INSOMNIA AND FATIGUE AFTER TRAUMATIC BRAIN INJURY

INSOMNIA AND FATIGUE AFTER TRAUMATIC BRAIN INJURY

A CBT Approach to Assessment and Treatment

MARIE-CHRISTINE OUELLET
School of Psychology, Université Laval, Québec, QC, Canada;
Center for Interdisciplinary Research in Rehabilitation and Social Integration (CIRRIS),
Québec, QC, Canada

SIMON BEAULIEU-BONNEAU
School of Psychology, Université Laval, Québec, QC, Canada;
Center for Interdisciplinary Research in Rehabilitation and Social Integration (CIRRIS),
Québec, QC, Canada

JOSÉE SAVARD
School of Psychology, Université Laval, Québec, QC, Canada;
CHU de Québec-Université Laval Research Center, Québec, QC, Canada;
Université Laval Cancer Research Center, Québec, QC, Canada

CHARLES M. MORIN
School of Psychology, Université Laval, Québec, QC, Canada;
CERVO Brain Research Centre, Québec, QC, Canada

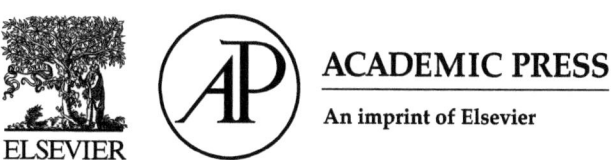

ACADEMIC PRESS
An imprint of Elsevier

Academic Press is an imprint of Elsevier
125 London Wall, London EC2Y 5AS, United Kingdom
525 B Street, Suite 1650, San Diego, CA 92101, United States
50 Hampshire Street, 5th Floor, Cambridge, MA 02139, United States
The Boulevard, Langford Lane, Kidlington, Oxford OX5 1GB, United Kingdom

Notices
Knowledge and best practice in this field are constantly changing. As new research and experience
broaden our understanding, changes in research methods, professional practices, or medical
treatment may become necessary.

Practitioners and researchers must always rely on their own experience and knowledge in
evaluating and using any information, methods, compounds, or experiments described herein.
In using such information or methods they should be mindful of their own safety and the safety of
others, including parties for whom they have a professional responsibility.

To the fullest extent of the law, neither the Publisher nor the authors, contributors, or editors,
assume any liability for any injury and/or damage to persons or property as a matter of products
liability, negligence or otherwise, or from any use or operation of any methods, products,
instructions, or ideas contained in the material herein.

British Library Cataloguing-in-Publication Data
A catalogue record for this book is available from the British Library

Library of Congress Cataloging-in-Publication Data
A catalog record for this book is available from the Library of Congress

ISBN: 978-0-12-811316-5

For Information on all Academic Press publications
visit our website at https://www.elsevier.com/books-and-journals

Publisher: Nikki Levy
Acquisition Editor: Nikki Levy
Editorial Project Manager: Barbara Makinster
Production Project Manager: Bharatwaj Varatharajan
Cover Designer: Mark Rogers

Typeset by MPS Limited, Chennai, India

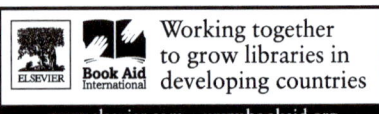

Contents

Preface   xi

Part I
ESSENTIAL BACKGROUND

1. Insomnia and Fatigue Following Traumatic Brain Injury:
Prevalence, Correlates Evolution, and Treatment Options   3

Traumatic Brain Injury: A Brief Overview   3
    Definition and Epidemiology of Traumatic Brain Injury   3
    Care Trajectories and Prognosis and After Traumatic Brain Injury   5
    Common Sequelae Following Traumatic Brain Injury   8
Post—TBI Insomnia   14
    Nature and Prevalence of Insomnia After Traumatic Brain Injury   14
    Etiology of Post—TBI Insomnia   15
    Evolution of Insomnia   18
    Potential Impacts of Post—TBI Insomnia   20
    Treatment Options for Post—TBI Insomnia   22
Post—TBI Fatigue   29
    Nature, Prevalence, and Impacts of Post—TBI Fatigue   29
    Etiology and Correlates of Post—TBI Fatigue   30
    Evolution of Post—TBI Fatigue and Its Relation to Traumatic Brain Injury
    Severity   33
    The Phenomenology of Post—TBI Fatigue   36
    Treatment Options for Fatigue   37
Interaction Between Insomnia and Fatigue   40
References   41

2. Assessment of Insomnia and Fatigue Following Traumatic
Brain Injury   61

Assessment: A Dynamic Process   61
What to Assess   62
    History, Nature, and Manifestations of Insomnia and Fatigue Symptoms
    Since the Injury   62
    Impact of Insomnia and Fatigue Symptoms on Evolution of Brain Injury
    Condition/Adaptation   63
    Habitual Sleep—Wake Schedule   63

Medications and Treatments	64
Lifestyle and Environmental Factors	64
Screening for Other Sleep Disorders	65
Screening for Psychopathology	65
Types of Assessment	66
Clinical Interviews	66
Diaries	67
Questionnaires	70
Objective Measures	71
Assessing the Patients' Readiness for Intervention	72
Assessment Tools Suggested in This Manual	74
References	74

3. CBT Interventions for Insomnia and Fatigue in the Context of TBI: Rationale, Adaptations, and Clinical Challenges   77

General Cognitive–Behavioral Therapy Treatment Components	77
Fostering a Self-Management Approach	77
Establishing Effective Self-Monitoring	79
Cognitive–Behavioral Therapy Components Specifically for Post–TBI Insomnia	82
Psychoeducation About Normal Sleep, Sleep After Traumatic Brain Injury, and Insomnia	82
Sleep Hygiene Education	83
Restriction of Time in Bed: Limiting Time Spent in Bed to Actual Sleeping Time	83
Stimulus Control: Recreating a Time and Space for Sleep	86
Brief Cognitive Therapy for Insomnia: Working on Unhelpful Thoughts, Beliefs, and Attitudes About Sleep and Insomnia	87
Cognitive–Behavioral Therapy Components Specific to Post–TBI Fatigue	90
Psychoeducation About Fatigue After Traumatic Brain Injury, and Health Habits Influencing Energy Levels	90
Increasing Self-Awareness of Energy Levels and Signs of Fatigue	91
Activity Management or "Pacing" for Fatigue	92
Working on Attitudes About Fatigue	94
Additional Components	95
Encouraging Graded Physical Exercise	95
Stress and Worry Management	96
Involving a Family Member	96
Clinical Challenges in the Context of Traumatic Brain Injury	98
Cognitive Impairment	98
Behavioral Particularities	99
Physical Impairment	100
Polypharmacy and Sleep Medication	100
Symptoms of Anxiety and Depression	101
Issues With Adherence and Motivation	101
References	102

Part II

PRACTICAL TOOLS

4. Assessment Tools for Post-TBI Insomnia   107

Overview   107
DSM-5 Diagnostic Criteria for an Insomnia Disorder   108
Clinical Interview on Insomnia Following Traumatic Brain Injury—Full Version   109
Clinical Interview on Insomnia Following Traumatic Brain Injury—Short Version   118
Sleep Diary   120
Sleep Diary (Full Version)—Example and Instructions   121
Sleep Diary—Short Version   122
Sleep Diary—Analysis   123
How to Compute Sleep Efficiency   124
Insomnia Severity Index (ISI)   126
Insomnia Severity Index (ISI)—Scoring and Interpretation   128
Dysfunctional Beliefs and Attitudes about Sleep (DBAS)   129
Dysfunctional Beliefs and Attitudes about Sleep (DBAS)—Scoring and
Interpretation   134
Case Conceptualization Summary for Post-TBI Insomnia   135

5. Assessment Tools for Post-TBI Fatigue   137

Overview   137
Proposed Diagnostic Criteria for TBI-Related Fatigue   138
Clinical Interview on Fatigue Following Traumatic Brain Injury   139
Energy/Activity Diary   143
Energy/Activity Diary—Example and Instructions   145
Energy/Activity Diary—Analysis   146
Multidimensional Fatigue Inventory (MFI)   147
Multidimensional Fatigue Inventory (MFI)—Scoring and Interpretation   148
Fatigue Severity Scale (FSS)   150
Fatigue Severity Scale (FSS)—Scoring and Interpretation   151
Fatigue Numerical Rating Scale   152
Fatigue Barometer   153
Case Conceptualization Summary for Post-TBI Fatigue   154

6. Intervention Tools for Post-TBI Insomnia   157

Overview   157
Clinician Guides:
    Overview of Interventions Strategies for Post-TBI Insomnia   159
    Establishing Effective Self-Monitoring With the Sleep Diary   164
    Presenting Basic Information on Insomnia   169
    Presenting Basic Information on Sleep   175
    Presenting Basic Information on Sleep Hygiene   179
    Stimulus Control: Recreating a Time and Place for Sleep   183

Restriction of Time in Bed: Limiting the Time Spent in Bed to Actual
Sleeping Time   189
Brief Cognitive Therapy: Promoting Beliefs and Attitudes That are Conducive
to Sleep   198
Motivational Strategies When Encountering Resistance   207
Clinical Challenges and Solutions to Adapt CBT for Insomnia to the
Context of TBI   208
Patient Handouts:
Self-Management of Insomnia   160
Helping a Family Member or Friend Manage Insomnia
(For Significant Others)   162
An Essential Tool: The Sleep Diary   167
Sleep Following a Traumatic Brain Injury   170
What is Chronic Insomnia and How Common Is It?   171
What Causes Insomnia?   172
Factors Which Perpetuate Insomnia   173
How Sleep is Produced   176
Stages of Sleep and Sleep Cycles   178
Sleep Hygiene: Maintaining Lifestyle Habits That Promote Good Sleep   180
Recreating a Time and Place for Sleep   185
Limiting the Time Spent in Bed to Actual Sleeping Time   194
My Motivating Activities   199
Beliefs and Attitudes That Promote Good Sleep   200
Strategies for Better Management of Worries When Going to Bed or During
Nighttime Awakenings   204

7. Intervention Tools for Post-TBI Fatigue   **211**

Overview   211
Clinician Guides:
Overview of Intervention Strategies for Post-TBI Fatigue   213
Establishing Effective Self-Monitoring With the Energy/Activity Diary   219
Presenting Basic Facts About Fatigue and Understanding the Vicious Circle
of Fatigue and the Benefits of Better Energy Management   223
Understanding the Connection Between Lifestyle Habits and Fatigue   228
Improving Self-Perception of Signs of Fatigue   231
Understanding Energy Fluctuations and the Activity–Fatigue Connection   234
Counteracting Inactivity by Gradually Increasing Activity Level and Planning
Rest Periods   241
Strategies to Adapt Activities in Order to Manage Energy Levels Effectively   246
Promoting Attitudes and Expectations for Good Energy Management   257
Gradually Increasing Physical Exercise   263
Patient Handouts:
Self-Management of Energy   215
Helping a Family Member or Friend Manage Fatigue (for Significant Others)   217
An Essential Tool: The Energy/Activity Diary   221
Fatigue Following a TBI   225
The Vicious Circle of Fatigue   226

The Positive Cycle of Effective Energy Management   227
Healthy Habits to Optimize Energy   230
Recognizing the Signs of Fatigue   233
Understanding the Activity–Fatigue Connection (Example)   235
Understanding the Activity–Fatigue Connection   237
Identifying Sources of Energy and Fatigue   238
Different Ways to Rest   243
Recommendations Concerning Naps and Rest Periods   245
Adapting Activities to Minimize Fatigue   248
Identifying High-Risk Situations   253
Maintaining a Balance Between Different Types of Activities   258
Maintaining Realistic Expectations About My Energy Levels   260
Reintegrating Avoided Activities and Integrating New Activities 261
Increasing Physical Activity to Fight Fatigue   265

8. Detailed Treatment Plan   269

Overview   269
Overview of Treatment Session Outlines   271
Treatment Session 1   272
Treatment Session 2   274
Treatment Session 3   276
Treatment Session 4   278
Treatment Session 5   280
Treatment Session 6   282
Treatment Session 7   284
Treatment Session 8   286

Index   287

Index   287

Preface

Often referred to as a silent epidemic, traumatic brain injury (TBI) can result in significant disability and major costs for patients, families, and society. Among the sequelae of TBI, fatigue and sleep disturbances, particularly insomnia, are particularly prevalent and persistent, and they can significantly impact quality of life. The complex interplay between pathophysiological processes, psychological factors, and social stressors contributes to the development of insomnia and fatigue following TBI, and requires thorough assessment and careful planning of management strategies. Despite their striking prevalence, the scientific interest for the etiology, assessment, and treatment of sleep—wake disturbances following TBI has only emerged in the last 10—15 years. Researchers and clinicians are increasingly stressing the importance of paying closer attention to post-TBI sleep and fatigue problems, realizing their potential impacts on functional recovery and long-term functioning after a brain injury.

There is a very strong evidence base for the treatment of insomnia with nonpharmacological interventions, particularly cognitive—behavioral therapy (CBT). CBT induces long-lasting benefits, not only on sleep quality and energy levels, but also on mood and motivation, which are key factors for optimal social participation. In addition, CBT for insomnia may be administered by a variety of professionals, including psychologists, neuropsychologists, occupational therapists, and nurses, and can be offered either as a stand-alone intervention or in combination with medication. CBT is now established as the first-line treatment for either primary insomnia (i.e., unrelated to other medical conditions) or insomnia comorbid to a medical or psychiatric condition. The goal of CBT is to induce durable changes in behaviors and attitudes through the development of self-management skills that will continue to be used by patients well beyond therapy sessions. Evidence is now emerging that CBT for insomnia is both feasible and efficacious with persons having sustained TBI. Our goal was thus to increase accessibility to this type of therapy for patients with TBI.

Although post-TBI sleep disturbances have been the object of growing research, interventions for post-TBI fatigue remain critically under-researched despite the far-reaching impacts of chronic fatigue on TBI patients' everyday life. Anchored in CBT principles that have been used successfully in other clinical populations and by clinicians for many years, we gathered tools to guide patients toward self-management of energy and fatigue. We believe it is essential to empower patients to become experts of their own fatigue and energy levels. Such mastery is built through self-observation and experimentation in one's everyday activities, which implies its share of trials, errors, successes, and setbacks. Clinicians can significantly contribute to guide these processes, and can help patients learn to live with residual fatigue while augmenting their capacity to reengage in valued activities or to explore new interests and roles, thus contributing to optimizing their quality of life and social participation.

The journey of the development of the present manual started in 2001 with the elaboration of clinical research protocols to study the nature and prevalence of insomnia and fatigue following TBI, and to evaluate the efficacy of CBT in this population. This led to a fruitful and ongoing collaboration between the authors of this manual. Since its beginnings, this work was largely based on the seminal work of Charles M. Morin (Full Professor, Université Laval, Québec, Canada) in the field of insomnia, to which was integrated expertise linked to the psychological aspects of brain injury (Ouellet, Beaulieu-Bonneau), and to the adaptation of CBT for insomnia for individuals with comorbid medical conditions (Savard). Our initial work (2001–07) led to the publication of large-scale surveys pertaining to the nature, prevalence, and correlates of insomnia and fatigue after mild-to-severe TBI, and to the first evidence that CBT could be adapted and effective to improve these issues in persons with brain injury.

The present manual is based not only on our research but also on multiple collaborations, which blossomed throughout the years. From the moment our research and clinical interests emerged, strong ties were developed with the Traumatic Brain Injury Rehabilitation Unit of the *Institut en déficience physique de Québec-IRDPQ* (now part of the *Centre intégré universitaire de santé et de services sociaux de la Capitale Nationale*), which is the main rehabilitation center for Eastern Québec offering both inpatient and outpatient rehabilitation services to individuals with acquired brain injury. Initially, we worked closely with neuropsychologists Catherine Truchon, Jean-François Cantin, and occupational therapist Claire Landry who had developed a specific interest relative to post-TBI fatigue. Despite the paucity of research, evaluations and interventions to manage fatigue issues were underway every day in the rehabilitation center and these clinicians had developed precious clinical expertise to guide our clinical research projects. It quickly became clear that it was essential to capture this expertise in a perennial form that would foster research in the field, contribute to knowledge transfer between clinicians, and ensure training of the next generation of clinicians.

In 2007 Jean-François Cantin formalized a Fatigue Committee that worked and evolved between 2007 and 2014, integrating the clinical expertise of occupational therapists Nancy Turcotte and Julie Lessard, and neuropsychologists Isabelle Potvin, Julie Dionne, Guylaine Duchesneau, and Nathalie Boutin. As clinical researchers, we were also part of this committee. This group also gained the support of decision makers and professionals including Lise Binet, Johanne Trahan, Anne Bourassa, Nancy Benoit, Monique Delisle, and Debbie Furlotte. The Committee embarked on a rigorous and structured process to collect the evidence from research, existing tools to support fatigue management (in French or English), and existing clinical expertise. Qualitative data were collected to elicit concrete recommendations from clinicians with experience in fatigue management, research results were gathered from the literature, and a variety of tools from the fields of stroke, multiple sclerosis, and chronic fatigue were consulted. After many years of collaboration between our research team and this committee, our efforts translated into a first tangible tool, *Le guide de l'énergie* (Cantin et al., 2014), which compiled tools for fatigue management for populations in rehabilitation at large. This document was made available freely on the internet via the IRDPQ's website.

In parallel, our research team received a knowledge translation grant from the *Fonds de Recherche Québec-Santé* for the elaboration of a manual specific to the TBI population, the *Manuel d'évaluation et d'intervention pour l'insomnie et la fatigue après un traumatisme craniocérébral* (Ouellet, Beaulieu-Bonneau, Savard, & Morin, 2015). The elaboration of the latter was supported by an advisory board composed of additional researchers, in particular Catherine Wiseman-Hakes and the late Joshua Cantor, translation expert Marie-Eve Lamontagne, also supported by Anne-Sophie Allaire, and by key members of a knowledge translation support organization, the *Centre de liaison sur l'intervention et la prévention psychosociales* (Stéphanie Taillon, Laurie Prud'homme, Mathieu Massejolicoeur). In the 5 years of this project, we led a province-wide survey of needs in terms of knowledge and tools for the evaluation and management of post-TBI insomnia and fatigue (94 rehabilitation professionals across 6 rehabilitation centers), and involved 12 clinician-champions in the testing of our material to ensure its usability. Clinicians who tested the material or offered their clinical expertise included Nathalie Boutin, Anick Charbonneau, Carole Cressaty, Julie Dionne, Guylaine Duchesneau, Julie Lessard, Geneviève Léveillé, Julie Ouellet, Isabelle Potvin, Teresa Testa, Martin Thériault, and Nancy Turcotte. We would also like to thank Jean-Philippe Savalle, a TBI survivor, whose website inspired some exercises and tools for fatigue management, Joachim Lépine who translated part of the material from French to English, and Mélanie Leblanc and Myriam Giguère for their coordination skills. In its final form the French manual included practical, ready-to-use tools, and was disseminated to 19 French-speaking rehabilitation facilities in the province of Québec and beyond, and is freely available on the Internet.

This book includes practical tools that have emerged from these previous projects and collaborations. As such, the nonlinear path toward this manual was shared by a number of wonderful people dedicated to the well-being of people who have sustained a brain injury. We hope that through this work, we will succeed in bringing this collective effort closer to those who can benefit from these interventions.

References

Cantin, J.-F., Ouellet, M.-C., Turcotte, N., Lessard, J., Potvin, I., Boutin, N., & Duchesneau, G. (2014). *Le guide de l'énergie: vers une meilleure gestion de la fatigue.* Québec: Institut de réadaptation en déficience physique de Québec. Available from https://www.ciusss-capitalenationale.gouv.qc.ca/publications-de-lirdpq/guide-de-lenergie-vers-une-meilleure-gestion-de-la-fatigue.

Ouellet, M.-C., Beaulieu-Bonneau, S., Savard, J., & Morin, C. (2015). Manuel d'évaluation et d'intervention pour l'insomnie et la fatigue après un traumatisme craniocérébral. Available from http://www.cirris.ulaval.ca/fr/insomnie-et-fatigue-apres-un-traumatisme-craniocerebral.

PART I

ESSENTIAL BACKGROUND

Insomnia and Fatigue Following Traumatic Brain Injury: Prevalence, Correlates Evolution, and Treatment Options

TRAUMATIC BRAIN INJURY: A BRIEF OVERVIEW

Definition and Epidemiology of Traumatic Brain Injury

Traumatic brain injury (TBI) is a major public health issue with far-reaching consequences for the injured persons, their families, and the community. Every year in the United States, at least 1.7 million individuals sustain a TBI, and between 2.5 and 6.5 million people live with the impacts of such an injury (Faul, Xu, Wald, & Coronado, 2010; Ragnarsson et al., 1999). The exact incidence and prevalence of TBI is difficult to establish because many persons do not consult after a mild TBI (or concussion), or because they access services outside hospitals and are often not accounted for by epidemiological studies (e.g., a family physician, neuropsychologist, physical therapist). In only a 1-year span, in 2013, the Center for Disease Control in the United States reported 2.8 million TBI-related visits to an emergency department (ED), hospitalizations, or deaths (Taylor, Bell, Breiding, & Xu, 2017).

Individuals who sustain TBI can experience temporary or permanent difficulties in multiple domains of functioning, including cognition (e.g., problems with attention, memory, executive functions), physical health (e.g., motor limitations, pain, sensory deficits), psychological health (e.g., depression, anxiety, substance misuse), and social life (e.g., unemployment, loss of driving license, marital issues, reduction of social support) (Silver, McAllister, & Yudofsky, 2005). These different domains of functioning all mutually influence each other, for example, pain increasing cognitive or emotional problems and vice versa. The severity, duration, and persistence of TBI-related consequences will depend on a plethora of factors including the severity of the injury, the localization of the brain damage, various preinjury characteristics (education, cognitive and psychological resources, personality factors, cognitive reserve, medical, psychiatric, and substance use history), and postinjury factors (medical complications, psychosocial stressors, health issues, coping strategies, and personal resources).

TBI is incurred when there is "an alteration of brain function (e.g., loss of or decreased level of consciousness, loss of memory for events immediately before—retrograde amnesia—or after—posttraumatic amnesia—the injury), or other evidence of brain pathology (i.e., visual, neuroradiological, or laboratory confirmation of damage to the brain), caused by an external force (e.g., acceleration/deceleration movement of the brain, head being struck by or striking an object, foreign body penetrating the brain)" (Menon, Schwab, Wright, & Maas, 2010). The majority of TBIs are blunt injuries (as opposed to penetrating injuries) and the two most frequent causes of TBI are motor vehicle accidents and falls. At the time of the injury, multiple pathophysiological events may occur, including primary damage (i.e., contusions, lacerations, hematomas, axonal injury). Other pathophysiological cascades follow the initial injury and are thus called secondary damage, involving various processes that can cause further damage to cerebral tissue, such as inflammation, ischemia, elevated intracranial pressure, abnormal neurotransmitter release, or hormonal changes. Because the brain undergoes strong rotational forces within the skull, stretching or twisting of axons can occur, causing a phenomenon known as diffuse axonal injury in various areas of the brain. Damage to the frontal and temporal lobes is frequent because of "coup and/or contrecoup" forces (when the brain bounces back and forth or sideways within the cranium). TBI seldom affects a single area of the brain and often leads to diffuse damage which explains the multitude of physical, social, cognitive, and psychiatric symptom presentations postinjury. Cerebral atrophy has been observed up to a year post-TBI suggesting that the brain continues to reorganize over many months (Sidaros et al., 2009).

The severity of TBI is generally evaluated as mild, moderate, or severe according to several criteria including the initial level of consciousness of the person at the time of injury, usually evaluated with the Glasgow Coma Scale (a score of 13−15 usually indicative of mild TBI; 9−12: moderate; 8 or less: severe), the duration of loss of consciousness (0−30 minutes: mild; 30 minutes to 24 hours: moderate; and >24 hours: severe), the duration of posttraumatic amnesia (<1 day: mild; 1−7 days: moderate; and >7 days: severe), and neurological and neuroimaging results. The majority of TBIs are mild (80%−90%), 5%−10% are moderate, and 5%−10% are severe (Cassidy et al., 2004; Tagliaferri, Compagnone, Korsic, Servadei, & Kraus, 2006). Males are twice more likely than females to sustain a TBI. There are major incidence peaks related to age in young children (0−4 years) mainly due to falls, adolescents and young adults (15−24 years) caused mainly by motor vehicle accidents, and older adults (>75 years) again due to falls (Faul et al., 2010). Other risk factors for TBI include substance misuse, lower socioeconomic status, lower education, unemployment, and having a psychiatric history (Bruns & Hauser, 2003).

Care Trajectories and Prognosis and After Traumatic Brain Injury

Mild Traumatic Brain Injury

Many individuals who sustain mild TBI do not consult for their injury and thus receive limited or even no medical attention. Some individuals will consult a health professional (e.g., primary care physician, physical therapist) after several days, weeks, or months, usually if there are persisting issues. Of those who visit an ED after a mild TBI, the majority are discharged shortly and are usually given information regarding signs necessitating a return to the ED or a medical evaluation, and recommendations for a gradual return to activities. Given the various potential trajectories of care, there probably is a great deal of variability in the information and recommendations provided to patients after mild TBI, and only a portion will receive specialized services, such as neuropsychology, physical or occupational therapy, or vocational rehabilitation services.

The prognosis after a first mild TBI (or concussion) is generally good, as the majority of individuals will be asymptomatic by 3−12 months postinjury (Losoi et al., 2016; van der Naalt, van Zomeren, Sluiter, & Minderhoud, 1999). The majority of patients (about 80%) will experience transient symptoms, such as headaches, dizziness, memory issues, irritability, or attention problems (Boake et al., 2005). While most of these symptoms will usually resolve, a nonnegligible portion of patients, between 15% and 30%, will experience some persisting symptoms in the physical, cognitive, or emotional realms (Carroll et al., 2014). For example, Barker-Collo et al. found that over the first year following mild TBI, the majority of patients improved on self-reported cognition, anxiety, mood, postconcussion symptoms, as well as neuropsychological measures (e.g., memory, complex attention, processing speed, executive function). However, at 6 months postinjury, more than 20% still presented poor performance on neuropsychological measures which were associated with mood problems, poor perception of cognitive outcomes, and residual postconcussion symptoms. At 12 months, this figure was still at 16%, suggesting that the recovery period after mild TBI may be longer than has been previously described (Barker-Collo et al., 2015). Another team found that at 6 months postinjury, 34% of a sample of persons with mild TBI still presented significant fatigue (Norrie et al., 2010). Persistent symptoms after mild TBI can be associated with functional decline, depression, impaired quality of life, and difficulty resuming work (Bombardier, Hoekstra, Dikmen, & Fann, 2016; Dahm & Ponsford, 2015a; Schiehser et al., 2015; Sirois et al., 2013).

It remains a major challenge to predict who will present persisting symptoms after mild TBI. A few prognostic factors include a history of preinjury mental health issues, delayed medical evaluation of the injury, and early postinjury anxiety or neuropsychological dysfunction (Silverberg et al., 2015; Stein et al., 2016; Waljas et al., 2014). Conversely, factors associated with remission of symptoms and return to work include absence of premorbid physical problems, low levels of pain, low levels of postconcussive and posttraumatic stress symptoms early after injury, higher education, absence of nausea or vomiting, and absence of additional extracranial injuries upon admission (Stulemeijer, van der Werf, Borm, & Vos, 2008). According to Hou et al. (2012), persons with similar injuries will react differently to the mild TBI because of cognitive–behavioral factors. In particular, they found that persistent symptoms were linked to negative illness perceptions and beliefs regarding the injury (e.g., attributing all symptoms to the TBI, believing that the symptoms would persist and have negative consequences, feeling a lack of control) and with all-or-nothing coping behavior (i.e., overdoing things when symptoms seem to be decreasing, then spending prolonged periods of time recovering once symptoms reoccur). These authors suggest that such cognitive–behavioral factors are amenable to intervention.

Prognosis can also be complicated by the number of mild TBIs sustained. Recuperation after a second concussion, for example, has been shown to be longer (Giza et al., 2013) and a history of repeated mild TBIs is linked to increased cognitive and mood issues (Horner, Selassie, Lineberry, Ferguson, & Labbate, 2008; Vynorius, Paquin, & Seichepine, 2016).

Moderate–Severe Traumatic Brain Injury

The trajectory of care following moderate or severe TBI usually involves admission to an intensive care unit and hospitalization (acute care), followed by inpatient rehabilitation, then outpatient rehabilitation, and finally community reintegration services (Cullen, Meyer, Aubut, Bayley, & Teasell, 2013). Following moderate-to-severe TBI, a period of posttraumatic amnesia of variable duration ensues, during which the patient is disoriented, often confused, and has major difficulty encoding new information. The emergence from posttraumatic amnesia constitutes a very important milestone in recovery as it is essential for the improvement of other cognitive functions. More so than other injury-related parameters, the duration of posttraumatic amnesia is in fact strongly correlated with long-term functional consequences, such as cognitive functioning or return to work. Compared to persons with mild TBI, recovery takes longer and permanent sequelae are more common after moderate–severe TBI. Patients will often go through several weeks or months of structured rehabilitation within a multidisciplinary team and receive intensive physical therapy, occupational therapy, psychology or neuropsychology, speech therapy, or exercise therapy, for example. In the inpatient context, patients' schedule, treatments, routines, and activities will be mainly dictated by the hospital or rehabilitation center staff. They might sometimes return home for short periods of time (e.g., a weekend) which will allow them to prepare themselves and their families to their return home and to the community. Outpatient services can be offered with various intensity and duration, for example, continuing physical therapy, neuropsychology, or vocational counseling.

Persons having suffered moderate or severe TBI can often live with permanent and significant cognitive deficits, as well as important behavioral changes. Furthermore, they may present a lack of awareness of their deficits or limitations (also known as *anosognosia*) (Prigatano, 2005; Richardson, McKay, & Ponsford, 2015). These sequelae can evolve over time as the person ages or goes through important life transitions. It is now widely admitted that moderate-to-severe TBI should be considered a chronic medical condition since many individuals live with the evolving sequelae of their injury for the rest of their life (Corrigan & Hammond, 2013; Masel & DeWitt, 2010). Significant help or services even after the rehabilitation phase are often necessary (Andelic et al., 2018). Indeed, although some issues may abate, others can actually worsen as the person ages. The following sections go into more detail about the possible consequences of TBI in different spheres.

Common Sequelae Following Traumatic Brain Injury

Physical Issues

TBI can lead to a wide array of physical consequences. These can include sensory impairments (visual disturbance, alterations in smell or taste, hearing loss), dizziness, hemiparesis, movement disorders, bladder and bowel issues, problems with swallowing or appetite, issues with sexuality, and alterations in balance and gait (Silver et al., 2005; Zasler, Katz, & Zafonte, 2012). About 15%–60% of patients with TBI present pituitary deficiencies (Kreber, Griesbach, & Ashley, 2016). About 10%–25% of individuals with moderate-to-severe TBI will develop posttraumatic epilepsy (Gupta et al., 2014). Unfortunately, because of the accident, TBI often cooccurs with injuries to other parts of the body, for example, fractured limbs. Compared to patients with orthopedic injuries without brain injury, having a TBI is associated with more physical injury, greater physical disability, and poorer functional status (Testa, Malec, Moessner, & Brown, 2005). The rate of chronic pain, especially headache, is very high among people who experience TBI (Martelli, Nicholson, & Zasler, 2013; Nampiaparampil, 2008). More than 50% of patients are estimated to have chronic pain, with headaches being the most commonly reported, followed by neck, shoulder, back, and upper limb pain (Khoury & Benavides, 2017). Headaches, which can affect between 30% and 90% of patients, are often chronic, can evolve into migraines (Moye & Pradhan, 2017), and can affect sleep or contribute to fatigue.

Cognitive Impairments

Cognitive impairments are the hallmark of TBI and can affect persons in the whole spectrum of injury severity. Many cognitive issues eventually resolve in patients with mild TBI (i.e., within 3 months) but the portrait can be much bleaker in the presence of a more severe injury, yet progress can be measurable even after 2 years (Trevena & Cameron, 2011). Difficulties with attention are extremely common (Morris, 2010) and can have an impact on concentration and one's capacity to stay on tasks and complete these satisfactorily. Information processing speed and efficiency is also often affected (Eslinger, Zappala, Chakara, & Barrett, 2012), and this difficulty is associated with marked mental fatigue (Johansson & Rönnbäck, 2014). Significant problems with short-term as well as long-term memory can be observed because of potential problems in various memory-related processes including acquisition and encoding of material into memory, and deficits in consolidation, retention, or retrieval of information (Morris, 2010). Language and communication difficulties can also be observed, some patients presenting slurred speech, word-finding problems, issues with oral or written comprehension, difficulty initiating or sustaining conversations, or speaking either too rapidly, too loudly, or too softly. Also quite common are deficits in executive functions, encompassing abilities for example in planning, organization, and perspective taking. Social cognition can also be affected, either subtly or significantly, and can encompass issues with the interpretation of social cues, recognition and understanding of emotions of others, and problems with generating appropriate responses to social cues (Allain, Togher, & Azouvi, 2018). The latter deficits can have a profound impact on social behavior.

Behavioral and Personality Changes

Although one's personality traits are usually expected to stay relatively stable over time, more severe TBIs can lead to changes in behavior and in the way the person interacts with the world. As such, significant others, for example, family members, friends, and coworkers, can perceive that the person has undergone an important "personality" change (O'Shanick, O'Shanick, & Znotens, 2011; Trevena & Cameron, 2011). For example, the patient may present decreased self-control and regulation, stimulus-bound behavior, emotional lability, decreased social perceptiveness, and difficulty to learn from social experience (the latter difficulties are linked to deficits in social cognition described earlier). An exacerbation of personality traits that were present prior to the injury can be also observed (O'Shanick & O'Shanick, 2005). Behavioral and personality changes are usually more marked in more severe injuries and these can significantly impact social relationships and it may result in alienation from others (O'Shanick et al., 2011), for example, if the person presents impulsivity, disinhibition, childish behavior (e.g., difficulties with turn-taking, sharing), or hyperverbosity (Cicerone & Maestas, 2014). Some individuals can also behave aggressively (physically or verbally), become irritable, or may be unpredictable (O'Shanick & O'Shanick, 2005). Kersel, Marsh, Havill, and Sleigh (2001a, 2001b) described the most common behavioral problems in a sample of 65 patients with severe TBI 6 months postinjury: irritability (49%), being more argumentative (44%), and increased anger (42%). These can be particularly difficult to manage for family members or caregivers and can affect patient−provider relationships.

Behavioral and personality changes may be less problematic in mild TBI, but it is common to see individuals who are more irritable or impatient, have mood swings, become more easily angry or aggressive, and these issues can cause frictions and tension with family members or friends. These problems can be exacerbated by fatigue or pain.

Social Network and Relationship Strain

TBI can have a significant impact on relationships, and the functioning of the couple or family can be impacted. According to different studies, between 33% and 78% of families report dysfunction after TBI (Gan, Campbell, Gemeinhardt, & McFadden, 2006; Testa, Malec, Moessner, & Brown, 2006). Couples may experience difficulties linked to changes in roles, loss of sexual intimacy, and decreased empathic communication, which are likely to create dyadic adjustments (Blais & Boivert, 2005). Some family members report an increase in responsibility for caring for the family, which can cause stress over time (Hoofien, Gilboa, Vakil, & Donovick, 2001). As a result, the risk of marital distress and separation following TBI is increased (Blais & Boivert, 2005; Kersel et al., 2001a, 2001b). TBI is also associated with decreases in social and leisure activities (Bier, Dutil, & Couture, 2009; Kersel et al., 2001a, 2001b). Higher levels of neurobehavioral dysfunction are expectedly associated with lesser social support (MacMillan, Hart, Martelli, & Zasler, 2002). Unfortunately, some studies suggest that social support tends to decrease over time after the injury (Morton & Wehman, 1995). This is of importance as social support is well known to serve as a protective factor for mental health in times of stress and psychosocial adversity.

Psychopathology

Between 31% and 65% of TBI survivors will meet the criteria for at least one psychiatric disorder over the first year postinjury. In fact, the first year after a TBI is known to be a critical time for the development of mental disorders (Alway, Gould, Johnston, McKenzie, & Ponsford, 2016). Depressive and anxiety disorders are the most frequent (Bryant et al., 2010; Diaz et al., 2012; Hesdorffer, Rauch, & Tamminga, 2009; Koponen, Taiminen, Hiekkanen, & Tenovuo, 2011; Whelan-Goodinson, Ponsford, Schonberger, & Johnston, 2010) and these are well known to be often accompanied by insomnia or fatigue. Compared to the general population, the rate of anxiety disorders is high in the first year but tends to normalize thereafter. Unfortunately, the rates of mood disorders are at least four times higher up to 5 years post-TBI. A history of a psychiatric disorder before the accident increases the risk of having a diagnosis post-TBI (Horner et al., 2008; Koponen et al., 2011). Nonetheless, it is important to note that 24%−45% of people without any previous psychiatric history will nonetheless develop a mental health problem in the first year postinjury (Bryant et al., 2010; Gould, Ponsford, Johnston, & Schonberger, 2011; Whelan-Goodinson, Ponsford, Johnston, & Grant, 2009).

Impacts on Daily Activities, Quality of Life, and Social Participation

Given the very large array of physical, behavioral, cognitive, and emotional challenges which can be brought about by TBI, daily activities, such as taking care of oneself, completing household chores, and fulfilling familial and work-related task, can become difficult, thus limiting the person's ability to engage in personally meaningful and valued activities (Toglia & Golisz, 2012). Quality of life and social participation are thus significantly affected after TBI (Polinder, Haagsma, van Klaveren, Steyerberg, & van Beeck, 2015). When comparing the physical and mental aspects of health-related quality of life, several studies have observed that the physical component tends to improve much faster than the mental component during the early months postinjury. Unfortunately, cognitive, emotional, and communication difficulties seem to persist over time, especially for moderate—severe injuries affecting quality of life and employment in the long-term (Grauwmeijer, Heijenbrok-Kal, Haitsma, & Ribbers, 2017; Grauwmeijer et al., 2018; Grauwmeijer, Heijenbrok-Kal, & Ribbers, 2014; Pagulayan, Hoffman, Temkin, Machamer, & Dikmen, 2008; Polinder et al., 2015). In a study by Dahm and Ponsford (2015c), employment rates were 54% at 1 year, 52% at 2 years, 65% at 5 years, and 64% at 10 years postinjury. Higher preaccident productivity and education level and younger age are predictive of return to work (Dahm & Ponsford, 2015c; Keyser-Marcus et al., 2002). It is also important to note that only 50% of people who have sustained moderate or severe TBI are fit to drive in the 5 postaccident years (Novack et al., 2010) which may be a factor limiting social, work-related, and recreational activities.

Impacts on Caregivers

Family caregivers, for example, spouses, parents, or children of the injured person, will very commonly compensate for the physical and cognitive limitations of their injured loved one. In fact, their help is often essential to the daily functioning of this person: they provide critical emotional and instrumental support to the person with TBI and significantly support the person's progress during rehabilitation and community reintegration (Lamontagne, Ouellet, & Simard, 2009; Lefebvre, Cloutier, & Levert, 2008). Both during and after rehabilitation, caregivers will take on new or increased responsibilities of support and care (Bayen et al., 2013; Degeneffe, 2001; Lamontagne et al., 2009; Sinnakaruppan & Williams, 2001). Although positive impacts also characterize the caregiving experience (e.g., a new intimacy, having a sense of personal growth, increased purpose, a sense of giving back), unfortunately, about half of the family members of adults with TBI suffer from psychological distress and one-third are significantly depressed (Doyle et al., 2013; Kreutzer et al., 2009). About 50% of caregivers of adult survivors experience significant burden and 40% have a lower than average quality of life (Doyle et al., 2013). When questioned about their needs, caregivers report that social well-being and emotional health are in fact their main concerns (Carlozzi et al., 2015).

Sleep—Wake Disturbances and Fatigue

Often mentioned among the physical consequences of TBI, sleep issues and fatigue are difficult to categorize into any given sphere of function because they involve physical, emotional, behavioral, cognitive, and motivational processes. They are also commonly viewed as problems secondary to other TBI-related issues. This may explain why they are often overlooked and have only recently received more scientific and clinical attention. Research is now quite clear that fatigue and sleep disturbances are among the most common consequences of TBI. These emerge within the complex interplay of preinjury, injury-related, and postinjury factors (see Fig. 1.1).

A variety of sleep-related symptoms and disorders are observed more frequently after TBI compared to the general population. This includes excessive daytime sleepiness, an increased need for sleep (especially early after the injury and/or in more severe injuries), sleep apnea, difficulties with circadian rhythms, and insomnia. Insomnia is the most frequent form of sleep disturbance observed after TBI because a large proportion of patients will report at least symptoms. In terms of prevalence of sleep disorders per se (disturbances significant enough to merit a diagnosis of a sleep disorder), hypersomnia (or excessive daytime sleepiness) is almost as frequent and should not be overlooked. Indeed, several sleep disorders (e.g., circadian rhythm sleep disorder, sleep apnea) could provoke symptoms which could be interpreted as insomnia. As such, careful evaluation and differential diagnosis is essential before initiating treatment for insomnia.

Post-TBI fatigue is also a widespread long-term complaint after TBI, much like it is a consequence of a plethora of other medical and neurological conditions (e.g., cancer, stroke, multiple sclerosis, encephalitis). Similarly to pain, fatigue is a subjective problem which has multiple dimensions (e.g., physical, mental, motivational, emotional). Fatigue thus affects the person's ability to participate in rehabilitation activities or to engage in valued activities and social roles. Like insomnia, fatigue can also interact or exacerbate other conditions which may be related to the injury or its aftermath, such as psychopathology, pain, or cognitive issues.

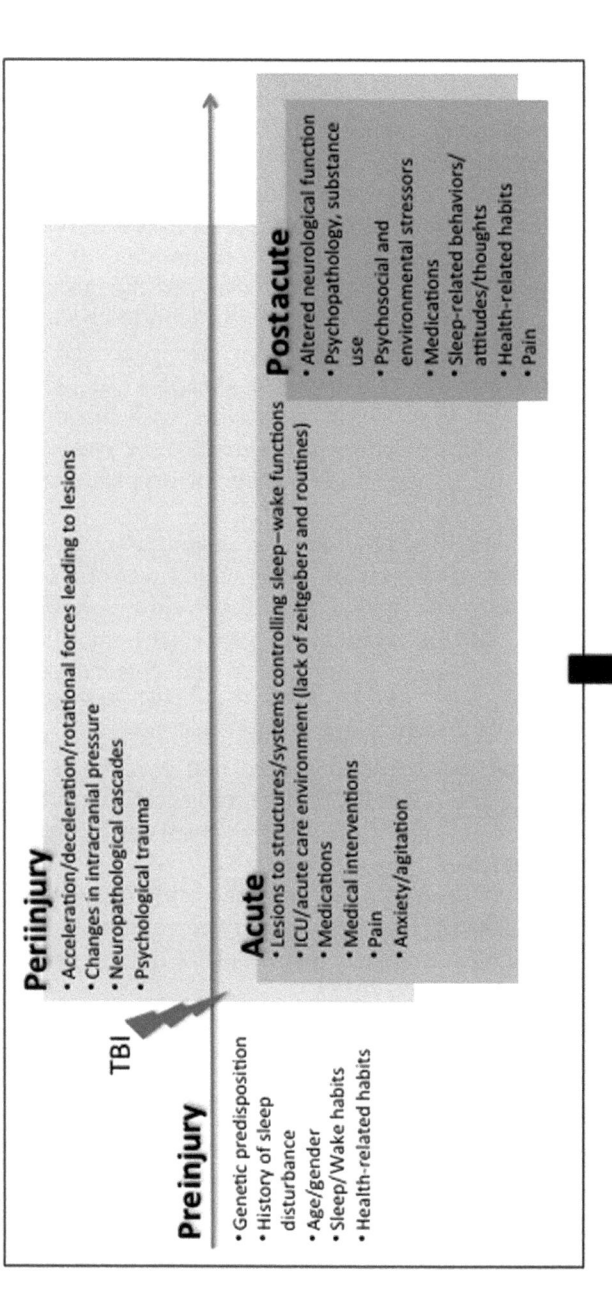

FIGURE 1.1 A model of potentially overlapping factors affecting sleep–wake patterns after traumatic brain injury. *Source: From Ouellet MC, Beaulieu-Bonneau S, Morin CM. Sleep–wake disturbances after traumatic brain injury. Lancet Neurol. 2015 Jul;14(7):746–57. https://doi.org/10.1016/S1474-4422 (15)00068-X. Review. PubMed PMID: 26067127. Reprinted with permission from Elsevier (The Lancet, 2015, Vol No. 14, 746–57).*

POST−TBI INSOMNIA

Nature and Prevalence of Insomnia After Traumatic Brain Injury

Insomnia is a very prevalent sleep issue following TBI. The most recent meta-analysis reports that 29% of TBI patients, regardless of the severity of the injury, meet the diagnostic criteria of an insomnia disorder, and about 50% have insomnia symptoms (Mathias & Alvaro, 2012). These numbers indicate that the occurrence of insomnia is at least two to three times higher after TBI than that seen in the general population. Indeed, between about 6% and 12% of adults in the general population meet criteria for an insomnia disorder per year and an additional 15%−20% report symptoms of insomnia (Morin et al., 2011; Ohayon, 2002; Roth et al., 2006). Risk factors associated with insomnia in the general population include suffering from a medical or psychiatric condition, being female, older age, and having an atypical work schedule.

One question which may arise is whether the insomnia observed after TBI is only a continuation of sleep difficulties which were present before the accident. We conducted a survey of 452 individuals having sustained mild-to-moderate TBI on average 8 years earlier. When using a combination of the diagnostic criteria of the International Classification of Sleep Disorders and the Diagnostic and Statistical Manual of Mental Disorders (DSM-IV), we found that 29% suffered from an insomnia syndrome. An additional 21% had symptoms of insomnia without fulfilling all the criteria. Of these, only 5.6% reported having sleep problems before the injury. In general, most participants reported that their sleep issues had appeared a few days (43.2%), a few weeks (14.4%), or a few months (28.8%) following the accident (Ouellet, Beaulieu-Bonneau, & Morin, 2006). These results were corroborated in a sample of mild TBI patients where less than 10% reported having preinjury sleep disturbances (Theadom et al., 2015).

Insomnia is characterized by subjective complaints of poor sleep quality or unsatisfactory sleep duration accompanied with difficulties initiating sleep (having problems falling asleep), frequent or prolonged periods of wakefulness during the night, or morning awakenings perceived as too early with an inability to go back to sleep. These problems occur despite having adequate opportunities to sleep and they are usually associated with clinically significant distress and/or impairment in daytime functioning. Indeed, beyond nocturnal symptoms, diurnal symptoms, such as fatigue, perception of impairment in cognitive functions (e.g., difficulties with attention, concentration, memory), and alterations in mood, may be present. The sleep difficulties must be present at least three nights or more per week and last for more than 3 months to meet the criteria for an insomnia disorder (American Academy of Sleep Medicine, 2014; American Psychiatric Association, 2013). The sleep difficulties should not be better explained by another sleep disorder.

Although the diagnosis of insomnia is based on subjective reports, there have been several sleep laboratory studies which have corroborated the subjective complaints of patients with TBI. A meta-analysis of 16 studies using polysomnography, a sophisticated objective measurement of sleep encompassing the monitoring of brain, muscle, and cardiac activity as well as eye movements, clearly reveals objective markers of altered sleep when persons with TBI are compared to healthy control groups: they have a reduced total sleep time, longer sleep onset latencies (time to fall asleep), increased time spent awake after sleep onset, and lower sleep efficiency which represents the time actually slept relative to the time spent in bed (Grima, Ponsford, Rajaratnam, Mansfield, & Pase, 2016).

Etiology of Post–TBI Insomnia

The causes of insomnia following TBI are complex, encompassing neurobiological factors, psychological processes, and factors linked to the environment.

Pathophysiology

One might first think of pathophysiological processes linked to brain damage which could explain sleep disturbances. There have been several studies which have indeed described links between sleep disturbances and various structural lesions or neurochemical or neuroelectric changes, but the underlying neuropathological processes remain obscure (Ouellet, Beaulieu-Bonneau, & Morin, 2015). One study found that the presence of sleep–wake disturbances was linked to abnormalities in white matter of the parahippocampal region (Fakhran, Yaeger, & Alhilali, 2013). Malfunctioning of the pineal gland and melatonin secretion has also been suggested as a potential cause of sleep disturbances after TBI (Yaeger, Alhilali, & Fakhran, 2014). Indeed, a reduced secretion and regulation of melatonin has been observed in both the acute and chronic phases post-TBI (Osier et al., 2017; Paparrigopoulos et al., 2006; Shekleton et al., 2010). Grima, Ponsford, St Hilaire, et al. (2016) found that when compared to healthy controls, persons with severe TBI had a 1.5 hour delay in the timing of dim light melatonin onset, as well as a 42% decrease of secretion of melatonin overnight. In more severe TBI, sleep–wake cycle disturbances, at least in the early phase after the injury, have been associated with abnormal hypothalamic function. Baumann et al. have found that persons with severe brain injuries show a loss in histamine and hypocretin wake-promoting neurons and a decrease in hypocretin-I, a neuropeptide involved in sleep/wake regulation (Baumann et al., 2009, 2005; Baumann, Werth, Stocker, Ludwig, & Bassetti, 2007; Valko et al., 2015), an anomaly also found in narcolepsy, which could explain the excessive daytime sleepiness frequently seen after TBI. Hypocretin-I levels tend to normalize by 6 months postinjury (Baumann et al., 2007).

The research to date has mainly elucidated the etiology of excessive daytime sleepiness and pertains more often to more severe injuries. The pathophysiological processes described earlier do not fully explain the development of insomnia symptoms in a large proportion of patients, especially in the longer term, up to months or years postinjury. This suggests that a variety of other factors may be at play, and as the person progresses into the subacute phase of recovery, it is thought that psychological factors may play a more important role in explaining post-TBI insomnia (Fichtenberg, Millis, Mann, Zafonte, & Millard, 2000; Ouellet, Beaulieu-Bonneau, Savard, & Morin, 2015).

Medication

Some medications prescribed to patients with TBI (e.g., corticosteroids, sedatives, analgesics, myorelaxants, anticonvulsants, antidepressants) can impact the architecture, quality, or quantity of sleep. Effects on sleep may vary depending on the dosage, timing, mechanism of function, and pharmacokinetics of the agent. Certain serotonin-selective reuptake inhibitors (SSRIs), for example, may decrease sleep efficiency (produce more awakenings, reduced total sleep time) and affect rapid eye movement (REM) sleep onset and duration (Ferguson, 2001).

Pain

Pain can cause somatic tension and arousal when a person is trying to fall asleep but can also impair the quality of sleep by introducing several microarousals during the different stages of sleep (Beetar, Guilmette, & Sparadeo, 1996; Moldofsky, 1989). Pain also interacts with anxiety and depressive symptoms and is often accompanied by *catastrophizing*, which involves rumination and exacerbation of feelings of helplessness related to one's condition (Khoury et al., 2013). The presence of one or more psychiatric conditions, such as depression, anxiety, and pain, increases the occurrence and severity of sleep problems (Fogelberg, Hoffman, Dikmen, Temkin, & Bell, 2012). Conversely, individuals with sleep complaints are more likely to develop headaches, depressive symptoms, and irritability (Chaput, Giguere, Chauny, Denis, & Lavigne, 2009). When sleep problems and pain become chronic after TBI, certain comorbid symptoms tend to appear or become chronic, including fatigue and depression (Beetar et al., 1996).

Psychopathology and Stress

Recovering from TBI will often involve a series of stressful events and can require major emotional adjustments to cope with new cognitive and/or physical limitations. Attempts to reintegrate different preinjury social roles (family life, work) may be difficult phases. These stressors can lead to increased cognitive and emotional arousal around bedtime or even during the night in the form of somatized tension, worrying, rumination, and anxiety (Morin, 1993; Ouellet, Savard, & Morin, 2004). Sleep disturbances in TBI can also be partly caused by comorbid psychopathology. Anxiety and depression levels are known to be clearly related to sleep disturbance, particularly insomnia severity, up to at least 2 years following TBI (Lowe, Neligan, & Greenwood, 2019; Ouellet et al., 2006; Parcell, Ponsford, Rajaratnam, & Redman, 2006). Depression is also an important predictor of insomnia in mild TBI (Farrell-Carnahan et al., 2015; Fichtenberg et al., 2000; Mollayeva, Shapiro, Mollayeva, Cassidy, & Colantonio, 2015). Conversely, insomnia seems to be a risk factor for the development of anxiety and depressive symptoms (Farrell-Carnahan et al., 2015). Rao et al. (2008) also described that insomnia appearing in within 3 months of the injury was closely tied to the appearance of an anxiety disorder, particularly generalized anxiety disorder.

Sleep-Related Habits

After TBI, one's habitual daily routines can be disrupted for long periods of time. For example, if unable to work, some individuals may lack the routine of regular arising time, getting ready for work, eating at regular times, and going to bed at relatively the same time. The lack of such zeitgebers (external cues which contribute to regulating the biological clock) may contribute to disrupt the sleep–wake cycle. Health-related habits, such as caffeine intake, alcohol or drug use, and eating habits, can also contribute to insomnia. Because of significant fatigue, many individuals will spend more time in bed, nap during the day, or take prolonged periods of rest. For example, in a sample of 452 individuals with mild-to-severe TBI surveyed on average 8 years postinjury, we found that 56% were still napping three to seven times per week (Ouellet & Morin, 2006). Napping and spending excessive time in bed are sleep-related habits which can actually contribute to desynchronize the sleep–wake cycle and thus may feed the sleep problem (Morin, 1993; Webb & Agnew, 1975).

Traumatic Brain Injury Severity

Insomnia complaints are present at all levels of severity of TBI (Farrell-Carnahan et al., 2015; Ouellet, Beaulieu-Bonneau, Savard, et al., 2015). Several studies suggest more insomnia complaints in individuals with milder injuries (Beetar et al., 1996; Farrell-Carnahan et al., 2015; Fichtenberg et al., 2000; Mahmood, Rapport, Hanks, & Fichtenberg, 2004; Ouellet et al., 2006; Shekleton et al., 2010; Viola-Saltzman & Watson, 2012). Variations of self-awareness of one's ongoing cognitive or behavioral issues are often pinpointed as one explanation for these results. Indeed, some individuals with moderate or severe TBI display impairments in self-awareness which can sometimes provide a buffer, to some extent, against psychological distress because they may not yet grasp the implications of their newly acquired limitations (Malec, Testa, Rush, Brown, & Moessner, 2007; McBrinn et al., 2008). Self-awareness is known to evolve, however, and psychological distress may develop as awareness increases through time, often as the person gradually tries to return to preinjury activities and roles. Individuals with milder injuries often return to the community setting and to their preinjury activities more rapidly compared to individuals with more severe injuries (who may require longer intensive rehabilitation services). A higher level of self-awareness coupled with this prompter return to activities may cause some individuals to feel more distress relative to their perceived residual issues after TBI (Demakis, Hammond, & Knotts, 2010). In turn, this can translate into more worrying and tension and impact on sleep quality.

Conversely, a few studies observed more insomnia in patient with more severe injuries (Cohen, Oksenberg, Snir, Stern, & Groswasser, 1992; Jain, Mittal, Sharma, Sharma, & Gupta, 2014) and several other studies have found no significant relationship between insomnia and severity of the injury (Castriotta et al., 2007; Parcell, Ponsford, Redman, & Rajaratnam, 2008; Rao et al., 2008; Theadom et al., 2015). In sum, insomnia can be an issue at all levels of the TBI severity spectrum.

Evolution of Insomnia

Sleep disturbances can emerge early after TBI. Sleep—wake patterns are usually disrupted in the first few days after the injury, especially after a moderate or severe TBI. It is well known that sleep is significantly disturbed while patients are treated in the intensive care unit, regardless of diagnosis: noise, light, pain, discomfort, frequent therapeutic or diagnostic procedures, anxiety, loneliness, and modification of routines can all contribute to sleep problems. Patients in the intensive care unit indeed have frequent awakenings, difficulty falling asleep, and sleep architecture can be significantly altered, for example, with a pronounced decrease or even eradication of deep or slow-wave sleep and REM sleep (Friese, Diaz-Arrastia, McBride, Frankel, & Gentilello, 2007; Gabor, Cooper, & Hanly, 2001). It is also very frequent to observe hypersomnolence in the first few days after TBI (Billiard & Podesta, 2013; Chiu, Chen, Chen, Chuang, & Tsai, 2013; Sommerauer, Valko, Werth, & Baumann, 2013). During the acute phase, there is a parallel trajectory between the normalization of sleep and recovery in consciousness and cognition. Sleep quality thus probably contributes to cerebral recovery (Duclos et al., 2017; Duclos et al., 2013; Duclos et al., 2016; Makley et al., 2009; Sherer, Yablon, & Nakase-Richardson, 2009).

Sleep disturbances can also emerge or be exacerbated during the subacute or more chronic phases after the injury. Important milestones, for example, attempting to return to work, can be accompanied by issues with sleep. Patients who had a history of sleep disturbance before the accident may experience a relapse or an increase in insomnia due to the injury, while those without any history of insomnia may develop it as a new condition (Rao et al., 2008). There are very few studies examining the longitudinal evolution of insomnia after TBI but if cross-sectional studies are examined together, insomnia remains high even several years postinjury (Beetar et al., 1996; Cohen et al., 1992; Farrell-Carnahan et al., 2015; Fogelberg et al., 2012; Jain et al., 2014; Ouellet et al., 2006; Perlis, Artiola, & Giles, 1997; Theadom et al., 2015). Theadom et al. (2015) examined sleep difficulties during the first year following a mild TBI. Of those reporting sleep difficulties at 1 month postinjury, 52% experienced an improvement in their sleep at the 6 months post-TBI mark, 17% reported that their sleep difficulties remained stable, and 31% unfortunately deteriorated further. Between 6 and 12 months, 38.9% saw a decrease in the quality of their sleep and for 16.2%, sleep difficulties remained stable (Theadom et al., 2015). In sum, according to this longitudinal study, for more than half of the participants, sleep difficulties remained chronic during the first year after TBI (Theadom et al., 2015). Another longitudinal study of insomnia following mild TBI was conducted by Jain et al. (2014) and found that most individuals experience insomnia symptoms in the first 3 months (63.41%) and a smaller proportion (36.57%) experience insomnia symptoms late, that is, between the third month and the first year after TBI (Jain et al., 2014).

Few data in the literature are available to describe the trajectories of insomnia in the long term. At 1 year post-TBI, the prevalence of insomnia symptoms is high, ranging between 30% and 46%, and this is much higher than that found in the general population, which is 10%–30% (Morin, LeBlanc, Daley, Gregoire, & Merette, 2006). To our knowledge, no longitudinal study has attempted to observe the evolution of insomnia over several years post-TBI according to TBI severity level. Fig. 1.2

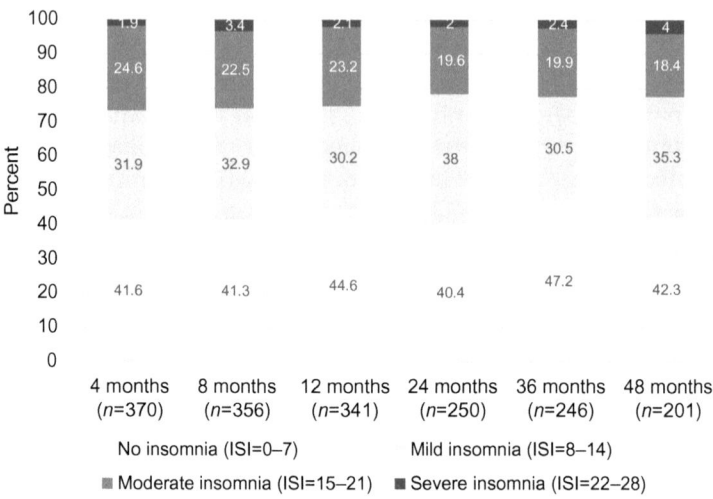

FIGURE 1.2   Distribution on scores of the Insomnia Severity Index (0–7 = no clinically significant insomnia; 8–14 = subthreshold insomnia; 15–21 = clinical insomnia-moderate severity; 22–28 = clinical insomnia-severe) according to time since injury in a prospective cohort of patients with mild (58.6%) and moderate–severe (41.2%) traumatic brain injury (mean age: 40.9 ± 15.04; 26% women) recruited at a Level I trauma center (Québec, Canada). *Source: Unpublished data (Gervais, Morin, Beaulieu-Bonneau, Ivers, & Ouellet, in preparation).*

presents yet unpublished and preliminary data from our team describing the evolution of insomnia symptoms up to 4 years post-TBI (4, 8, 12, 24, 36, and 48 months) with the Insomnia Severity Index (Morin, 1993). This was a cohort of adults having sustained either mild (58%) or moderate-to-severe TBI (42%) recruited at a Level I trauma center. Scores on the Insomnia Severity Index unfortunately remain quite stable over time with 30%–38% suffering from mild insomnia and another additional 22%–28% suffering from moderate-to-severe insomnia at any given time point. Individual trajectories of symptom severity over the first 4 years remain to be investigated, but clearly for a large proportion of individuals, post-TBI insomnia adopts a chronic course which calls for increased specific and specialized attention and care.

Potential Impacts of Post–TBI Insomnia

Using reports from health-care professional during rehabilitation for severe TBI, Worthington and Melia observed that 47.4% of their sample had disturbed sleep or problems arousal and in 65.6% of these, sleep–wake issues interfered significantly with rehabilitation interventions and daily activities (e.g., patients who were unable to stay awake during a therapy session or during an activity, patients missing their appointments because they stayed in bed). This suggests that sleep–wake issues can affect the person's capacity to effectively participate during rehabilitation therapies (e.g., occupational, physical, speech, or cognitive remediation therapies).

Few studies have examined the impact of post-TBI insomnia on specific neuropsychological measures. In a sample of 262 veterans with mild TBI, one team observed a relationship between shorter self-reported total sleep time the night prior to testing and memory performance (Waldron-Perrine et al., 2012). Further supporting the link between insomnia and cognitive performance, a few studies have shown that treating sleep disturbances (of various nature but including insomnia) may improve performance on neuropsychological tests, for examples, measures of attention, memory, processing speed, and language (Ruff, Ruff, & Wang, 2009; Wiseman-Hakes et al., 2013; Wiseman-Hakes, Victor, Brandys, & Murray, 2011).

The research is much clearer regarding the fact that insomnia complicates recovery and long-term outcomes after TBI. In patients on average 8 years postinjury, we found that more than half of the participants suffering from sleep disturbances (mainly insomnia) felt that their sleep problem interfered "a lot" or "extremely" with their mood, mental and social abilities, hobbies or main occupation, work or study, and their rehabilitation (Ouellet et al., 2006). In adolescents with mild TBI, sleep disturbances were found to be associated with a threefold increase in recovery time from the concussion. Suffering from insomnia at 1 or 2 years following moderate-to-severe TBI was also found to be associated with more functional limitations, greater reliance on others, and lower satisfaction with life (Cantor et al., 2012; Fogelberg et al., 2012). In adults, sleep–wake disturbances contribute to the chronicity of mood alterations and pain (Chaput et al., 2009). Theadom's team found that sleep quality as measured by the Pittsburgh Sleep Quality Index in the first 2 weeks after mild TBI was predictive of several functional parameters at 1 year postinjury including worse cognitive outcomes, lower productivity, and lower levels of social integration (Theadom et al., 2015). Recently, insomnia was found to be a clear predictor of disability in workers with mild TBI (Mollayeva, Mollayeva, Shapiro, Cassidy, & Colantonio, 2016). These results suggest that it may be important to address sleep disturbances early on after TBI, although it remains unclear whether interventions could have beneficial effects on long-term outcomes.

Although the links between post-TBI sleep–wake disturbances and physical health have received very little attention until now, a recent study found a 2.28-fold increased risk of suffering a stroke later on when insomnia was observed in comorbidity with TBI (Ao et al., 2017).

Treatment Options for Post—TBI Insomnia

Pharmacological Interventions

There is very little information on the safety and efficacy of pharmacological agents for insomnia in persons who have sustained a brain injury. When consulting recent clinical practice guidelines for rehabilitation and management of either mild or moderate—severe TBI (INESSS-ONF, 2016; ONF, 2018; VA/DoD, 2016), it is very clear that nonpharmacological interventions for insomnia are preferred to pharmacological interventions as the first line of treatment.

Benzodiazepine receptor agonists, which encompass benzodiazepines and the more recently developed "z-drugs" (i.e., zaleplon, zopiclone, zolpidem, eszopiclone), are often prescribed for insomnia in the general population. These are usually recommended only for short-term use (i.e., 4—6 weeks) or on an occasional basis (National Institutes of Health, 2005; Wilson et al., 2010). Other drugs are also used off-label for insomnia (e.g., antidepressants such as trazodone or doxepin, anticonvulsants such as gabapentin or tiagabine). Several authors call for great caution because certain medication will produce deleterious effects or can exacerbate issues related to the brain injury, for example, cognitive issues, fatigue, motor impairments, or dizziness. Some medications with anticholinergic effects (e.g., tricyclic antidepressants, diphenhydramine) can have negative effects on memory and attention and potentially lower the epileptic threshold. Flanagan, Greenwald, and Wieber (2007) advise to completely avoid benzodiazepines in the TBI population, because of potential aversive effects, such as dizziness, altered psychomotor skills, impaired memory, impacts on normal sleep architecture, and potential for abuse and dependence. Despite these potential adverse effect, one study showed that about 20% of TBI patients who were 9 years postinjury on average were making a long-term use of benzodiazepines or other hypnotic drugs, which goes against most clinical guidelines suggesting that these drugs should be used for a few months at most (Worthington & Melia, 2006).

Newer agents, such as z-drugs, seem to be preferred to manage insomnia after TBI, because they present a lower risk for tolerance, cause less withdrawal adverse effects, and seem associated with fewer daytime cognitive effects. Some authors still advise caution even with these newer agents since these may also have deleterious effects on cognition in the short or long term (Larson & Zollman, 2010). Chiu et al. (2015) documented an increased risk for dementia in TBI patients who used hypnotics. Those suffering from insomnia but not taking any sleep medication had a risk similar to those not suffering from insomnia after their injury.

Recently, in a sample of mild-to-severe TBI patients, Grima et al. (2018) showed that 2 mg of melatonin taken 2 hours before bedtime for 4 weeks resulted in a significant decrease in the Pittsburgh Sleep Quality Index score compared to a placebo group. These encouraging results were in addition corroborated by an increase in sleep efficiency as measured by actigraphy (a small watch-like device measuring sleep–wake activity). Furthermore, anxiety symptoms were also decreased and no adverse effects of melatonin were observed, suggesting its safety in patients with TBI.

Cognitive–Behavioral Therapy

Cognitive–behavioral therapy (CBT) is now considered the first line of treatment for insomnia; unfortunately, the access to therapy is still not optimal. A recent meta-analysis of 87 randomized controlled trials including at least one component of CBT for insomnia (e.g., sleep restriction, stimulus control, described later) included studies of patients with or without comorbid conditions (Ballesio et al., 2018). Significant effects of CBT are found for a variety of outcomes including sleep onset latency, time spent awake after sleep onset, sleep efficiency and quality, as well as scores on well-validated measures, such as the or the Insomnia Severity Index. Total sleep time is also improved, although to a lesser extent than other outcomes. Importantly, this meta-analysis shows that the efficacy of CBT is comparable in various samples, either with or without other medical or psychiatric conditions, and with younger or older adults. In terms of treatment modality, the authors found that face-to-face treatments which included at least four sessions were more effective than shorter or self-help interventions. CBT for insomnia also produces benefits on depressive symptoms (Ballesio et al., 2018).

CBT aims at modifying factors which perpetuate insomnia. Indeed, regardless of the cause of insomnia, individuals suffering from chronic insomnia most often present with cognitive and behavioral issues which often have an important role in the maintenance of insomnia over time, such as habits related to sleep, dysfunctional beliefs, and negative thought patterns (Espie, 2002; Harvey, 2005; Perlis & Buysse, 2011). Fortunately, these are often modifiable through therapy. For example, during the course of an illness causing significant pain, a person may develop acute sleep disturbances. Over the long term, however, the person may have developed habits, such as spending more time in bed trying to get rest, taking naps during the day to try to compensate for insomnia, or having irregular sleep–wake schedules. Sleep disturbances can also be accompanied by significant worrying about sleep and about the evolution of the medical condition per se, its impacts, and the impacts of poor sleep on the next day, and one's recovery. Even if the health condition may eventually resolve and the pain disappears, thoughts, attitudes, and habits can perpetuate insomnia due to conditioning factors.

Cognitive and behavioral interventions for insomnia include a variety of techniques, such as stimulus control, sleep restriction (or restriction of time in bed), cognitive therapy, sleep hygiene education, and relaxation or mindfulness-based techniques. CBT for insomnia will usually combine several of these therapeutic components. *Stimulus control* consists in a set of instructions which aim to weaken maladaptive conditioning processes by reassociating the bed, bedroom, and bedtime-related stimuli with sleep and relaxation rather than with tension, frustration, anxiety, and worrying about sleep (Bootzin, Epstein, & Wood, 1991). *Sleep restriction* (or restriction of time in bed) consists in establishing a "sleep window" which limits the time spent in bed to the average time that the patient actually spends sleeping, as assessed for example with a sleep diary for several days (Spielman, Saskin, & Thorpy, 1987). *Cognitive therapy* for insomnia is used to train the patient to identify and challenge unhelpful thoughts, beliefs, and attitudes about sleep (Morin, 1993). *Sleep hygiene education* is provided to inform the patient about links between health-related habits (e.g., diet, drug use, exercise) and sleep quality or duration. The influence of environmental factors (e.g., temperature, light, noise) on sleep is also examined and modifications are proposed as needed (Hauri, 1991). *Relaxation and mindfulness-based techniques* are used to lower physical and mental tension, for example, before bedtime.

Beyond the extremely solid empirical base of CBT for insomnia in a variety of patient populations, studies examining the efficacy of CBT for insomnia specifically in the TBI population are also emerging. Our team published the first preliminary evidence that CBT could be efficacious in patients with TBI when simple adaptations to the more "traditional" approach were made. We used the protocol developed by Morin (1993) which included 8 weeks of CBT and combined stimulus control, sleep restriction, cognitive therapy, and sleep hygiene education. The following adaptations were made: to ensure optimal comprehension and use of the diary, a period of close monitoring of sleep diary completion preceded the beginning of therapy during which patients were trained to use the diary, compile their information, and interpret it (this increases self-efficacy and empowerment); to optimize attention during sessions, shorter sessions and breaks were used as needed. To optimize encoding and retention of rationale of interventions and recommendations, information was repeated throughout sessions as needed and recommendations were presented orally as well as on paper (including figures/pictures). We added a fatigue management component (described further) including training to identify signs of fatigue, to plan and pace activities more adequately, incorporating rest periods, and exploring different ways to rest. A simplified cognitive therapy component was used. Indeed, instead of using Socratic questioning or other techniques requiring more insight or verbal abilities, the patients filled the Dysfunctional Beliefs and Attitudes About Sleep scale (Morin, Vallieres, & Ivers, 2007) which helped identify the major dysfunctional thoughts, beliefs, and attitudes to be addressed (e.g., "If I wake up during the night, I will not be able to function tomorrow"). A psychoeducational approach was used to challenge beliefs with short texts presented to the patient both orally and on paper. When dysfunctional thoughts were observed, the patient was guided toward alternative interpretations if unable to do so spontaneously, and alternative thoughts were noted in writing (e.g., on a cue card, on the sleep diary, or in the person's personal diary or planner). The cognitive therapy component also aimed at detecting and modifying thoughts related to the brain injury which may be distressing, for example, "My sleep problems will worsen my brain injury," "With this insomnia problem, I will never be able to return to work." Such thoughts may produce tension and worrying not only at bedtime or during nighttime awakenings but also during the day and contribute to increased performance anxiety related to sleep. Overall, the sessions were highly structured and patients brought their sleep diary and treatment material to every session. Patients were also encouraged to share their new comprehension or perspectives with their significant others. In fact, significant others were involved as possible to promote adherence, optimize motivation, and ensure comprehension of therapy recommendations. They were invited to the second or third session or contacted by phone.

We tested this protocol in a rigorous series of case studies (Ouellet & Morin, 2004, 2007) with patients having suffered mainly moderate and severe brain injuries (on average 2 years postinjury). Most patients (73%) showed significant reductions in total wake time and improved their sleep efficiency. This success rate was similar to those reported in samples of patients suffering from primary insomnia or insomnia comorbid to other medical disorders. Measures of general and physical fatigue were also reduced following treatment (but not *mental* fatigue unfortunately). Trends were also found for decreased depression and anxiety symptoms. Therapeutic gains were well maintained at a 3 months follow-up assessment. Of note, all of these patients had clinically significant cognitive deficits as documented by neuropsychological evaluations included in their medical files, and the majority had positive neuroimagery results indicating observable brain damage. The majority of patients had at least average intelligence (as assessed with a neuropsychological evaluation) but a few had low average or borderline levels of intelligence. Despite these characteristics, no patient had any major difficulty in understanding the rationale and nature of treatment recommendations, and all were able to learn how to use the sleep diary effectively. As such, this was the first demonstration that CBT for insomnia was feasible in patients with TBI (in fact at that time there was very little evidence in the literature of the efficacy of CBT for any type of psychological disturbance).

Recently, a rigorous randomized controlled trial evaluated the efficacy of CBT for insomnia and fatigue in a sample of mild-to-severe patients with TBI and stroke patients compared to a treatment-as-usual control (Nguyen et al., 2017). The treatment involved psychoeducation, reorganization of daily schedules, graded physical activity, cognitive restructuring, sleep interventions (stimulus control, sleep restriction procedures, relaxation), and strategies for managing physical and mental fatigue (e.g., pacing tasks, planning breaks). Clinically significant reductions of insomnia severity and overall improvement of sleep quality were observed in 70% of the CBT group compared to 27% in the control group. Fatigue was also reduced in 55% compared to 30% in the treatment-as-usual group and treatment gains were maintained 2 months posttreatment. Of note, these improvements in sleep and fatigue with CBT were paralleled a decrease in depressive symptoms. This research team also studied patient characteristics associated with better treatment responses (Nguyen et al., 2018). Premorbid intelligence, education, time since injury, and baseline severity of anxiety symptoms were not related to treatment outcomes. However, persons with more severe depression at baseline, younger individuals, and those with higher verbal memory scores had higher levels of improvement with therapy. This finding suggests that, at least in a mixed TBI–stroke sample, neuropsychological function, in particular memory, influences the efficacy of CBT for insomnia. The authors suggest that further adaptations to therapy should be considered with patients with memory issues, for example, by ensuring closer monitoring of their skill practice during therapy, or by modulating the intensity of therapy (planning shorter and more frequent sessions), or by reducing the content of therapy to fewer skills but repeating these skills more intensely (Nguyen et al., 2018).

In a recent case series, Lu, Krellman, and Dijkers (2016) used a preexisting four-session protocol of CBT for insomnia (Edinger & Carney, 2008) with three patients with mild, moderate, and severe TBI. The therapy included the use of a sleep diary, modification of poor sleep habits, psychoeducation, stimulus control and sleep restriction recommendations, use of thought records, and a "constructive worry" technique to manage presleep worrying. They made a few adaptations to the original protocol, for example, by providing handouts presenting homework (to promote learning and retention) and by helping patients to incorporate reminders of bedtime and arising time by programming alerts into their digital calendars or noting these into their traditional calendar. Although trends were observed, this four-session protocol was not sufficient to show clinically significant improvements in sleep, but interestingly, all participants showed clinically significant reductions in anxiety, two showed reductions in depression, and one showed a decrease in pain and fatigue (Lu et al., 2016). The authors conclude that CBT for insomnia may be an interesting treatment option to decrease anxiety and depressive symptoms.

Another research team recently made efforts to disseminate CBT for insomnia in the context of TBI by examining the potential efficacy of online interventions to improve sleep (Theadom et al., 2018). In a pilot randomized controlled trial with 24 individuals with mild or moderate TBI, they compared either online CBT to an online education condition. Their CBT intervention included sleep restriction, relaxation and mindfulness training and psychoeducation about sleep, and how environmental factors may affect sleep. In the control condition, participants were given information about brain injury, how the injury may affect sleep and fatigue and informed patients about the effects of exercise, environmental factors, diet, and substance use. Of note, the control group also received some guidance on how to establish a routine of periods of activity and rest. The study revealed that the CBT group had a more significant reduction in sleep disturbance compared to the control group. However, there was no significant difference between groups on objective sleep parameters (measured with actigraphy), quality of life, and cognitive functioning. It could be argued that in this study, the control group intervention was quite active. The team noted that two patients had problems completing the online program because of visual disturbances. Nonetheless, these results support the feasibility of online CBT to improve sleep in adults with mild-to-moderate TBI.

The research just reviewed was conducted with patients in the chronic phase after TBI. Still very little work has been done on cognitive–behavioral interventions in the acute phase after the injury. In a pilot study, De La Rue-Evans, Nesbitt, and Oka (2013) proposed a behavioral intervention to be implemented by nurses during acute rehabilitation. They obtained encouraging results. The program included making changes to the rehabilitation hospital environment, implementing systematic routines, providing sleep hygiene education to both nurses and patients, and using the principles of stimulus control. Nurses were encouraged to provide an environment more conducive to sleep (e.g., decrease noise levels, dim lights at night, open blinds before dawn, offer decaffeinated drinks later in the day or evening). They were also encouraged to keep patients active and awake throughout the day (maintaining a regular wake time, restricting naps) and to provide patients with an easily readable list of sleep-related recommendations. The research team found the intervention to be feasible and reported clinical benefits. Further research in the acute phase is necessary to better understand how early intervention can benefit patients in the longer term, for example, by diminishing the appearance or chronicization of sleep issues or by globally improving functional outcomes.

In sum, in addition to decades of research confirming the efficacy of CBT for primary insomnia and insomnia comorbid to medical or psychiatric conditions, evidence is now mounting that CBT for insomnia in various formats is not only feasible but also efficacious to improve sleep quality after TBI and probably has secondary positive impacts on associated factors, such as depression, anxiety, and fatigue.

Other Nonpharmacological Interventions for Post–TBI Insomnia

Vuletic et al. (2016) examined the effects of a problem-solving treatment (12 biweekly phone calls over a period of 6 months) compared to an educational module administered over the phone to active duty postdeployment service members who had sustained mild TBI. They not only taught traditional problem-solving skills but also proposed focused modules on either headache, insomnia, depression, or anxiety which patients could choose from. They found that this intervention significantly improved sleep quality, sleep onset latency, sleep efficiency, and sleep duration. The authors found that the intervention was particularly efficacious for sleep problems associated with pain.

A few studies have examined the effects of exercise on insomnia symptoms although in the context of interventions measuring a variety of cognitive or mood outcomes (Chin, Keyser, Dsurney, & Chan, 2015; Damiano, Zampieri, Ge, Acevedo, & Dsurney, 2016; Hoffman et al., 2010). Mixed results were found with only one study showing that 5 weekly sessions of 30 minutes of aerobic exercise for 8 weeks led to significant improvement on the Pittsburg Sleep Quality Index (Damiano et al., 2016).

Sinclair et al. tested the efficacy of blue light therapy for sleep disturbance, fatigue, and daytime sleepiness. They did not find any improvement for sleep quality, but fatigue and sleepiness did improve (Sinclair, Ponsford, Taffe, Lockley, & Rajaratnam, 2014). One pilot study found that acupuncture held promise to treat post-TBI insomnia compared to a treatment-as-usual condition. (Zollman, Larson, Wasek-Throm, Cyborski, & Bode, 2012). Patients treated with acupuncture were taking less sleep medication and had an improved perception of their sleep quality and better scores on some neuropsychological tests.

POST–TBI FATIGUE

Nature, Prevalence, and Impacts of Post–TBI Fatigue

Fatigue is a hallmark of many neurological conditions (e.g., stroke, multiple sclerosis, brain tumors, and other encephalopathies). Chaudhuri and Behan (2004) define it as a "failure to initiate and/or sustain attentional tasks and physical activities requiring self-motivation (as opposed to external stimulation)." Wylie and Flashman (2017) define fatigue as "A subjective lack of physical and/or mental energy that is perceived by the individual or caregiver to interfere with usual and desired activities. Perceptions of fatigue refer to subjective sensations of weariness, exhaustion, increasing sense of effort, or a mismatch between effort expended and actual performance."

Fatigue is often dichotomized in various ways: normal versus pathological, acute versus chronic, physical (e.g., loss of muscle strength) versus mental (e.g., difficulty focusing, mental fog, exhaustion, lower motivation), peripheral (relating to dysfunction of the peripheral nervous system) versus central (stemming from a dysfunction of the central nervous system) (Shen, Barbera, & Shapiro, 2006). After TBI, fatigue can probably be described as pathological, chronic, and central. Other types of fatigue have been suggested, such as emotional or stress fatigue. Fatigability is a term often used in the context of TBI and refers to the process fatigue build-up (magnitude or rate of change of fatigue) during a given task relative to a baseline performance (Wylie & Flashman, 2017). Although we often speak about fatigue as a one-dimensional construct (being significantly fatigued or not), post-TBI fatigue is in fact multidimensional encompassing physical, cognitive, emotional, and motivational dimensions (Cantor, Gordon, & Gumber, 2013; Ouellet, Beaulieu-Bonneau, & Morin, 2012; Wylie & Flashman, 2017). Mental fatigue seems to be an important type of fatigue felt following TBI, although more general and physical fatigue are also very prominent (Ouellet & Morin, 2006; Wylie & Flashman, 2017). Because fatigue is an elusive and subjective construct, it is difficult to measure and to investigate empirically. A few teams have attempted to measure fatigue objectively after TBI with neuropsychological tests (Ashman et al., 2008; Johansson & Ronnback, 2015; Ziino & Ponsford, 2006), but the use of self-reported measures probably best captures the subjective nature of the fatigue experience after TBI.

Many clinicians, patients, and researchers will agree that fatigue is a staggering consequence of TBI. Different studies have produced a wide range of prevalence rates, with some up to 80% of the samples (Belmont, Agar, Hugeron, Gallais, & Azouvi, 2006b; Englander, Bushnik, Oggins, & Katznelson, 2010; Mollayeva et al., 2014; Ouellet &

Morin, 2006). Most estimations of the prevalence of clinically significant fatigue following TBI range from 20% to 75% (Belmont, Agar, Hugeron, Gallais, & Azouvi, 2006a; Bushnik, Englander, & Wright, 2008a; Mollayeva et al., 2014; Olver, Ponsford, & Curran, 1996; Ouellet & Morin, 2006). Several researchers and clinicians have suggested that fatigue is *the* most common persisting symptom following TBI. In a longitudinal study of 141 patients up to 10 years after mainly moderate—severe TBI, Ponsford et al. (2014) found that fatigue was the most common complaint, with rates of 70% at 2 years postinjury, 60% at 5 years, and 57% at 10 years postinjury. More recently, the same team examined the rate of persisting symptoms on average 7 months postinjury this time following mild TBI, and fatigue was again the most common symptom (Ponsford et al., 2019).

Fatigue has tremendous impacts on injured persons and their families and communities. It contributes to overall disability, increased cognitive issues, and decreased quality of life (Bushnik, Englander, & Wright, 2008b; Cantor et al., 2008; Esbjornsson, Skoglund, & Sunnerhagen, 2013; Juengst, Skidmore, Arenth, Niyonkuru, & Raina, 2012; Ouellet & Morin, 2006; Stulemeijer et al., 2007). Speaking to its importance, it has been demonstrated that fatigue is the main reason for not being able to return to work after TBI (Dahm & Ponsford, 2015b; McCrimmon & Oddy, 2006).

Etiology and Correlates of Post—TBI Fatigue

Pathophysiology

The underlying causes of post-TBI fatigue are quite unclear and encompass a wide variety of factors. Because fatigue is a common consequence of a large array of neurological conditions, it certainly has a neuropathophysiological basis but which remains largely nebulous. Some authors have suggested that fatigue is linked to neuroendocrine abnormalities (which are common after TBI), dysfunctions in different neurological systems including the reticular activating system, the basal ganglia, and limbic system, and impaired excitability of the motor cortex (Bushnik, Englander, & Katznelson, 2007; Chaudhuri & Behan, 2004). Genetic factors (ApoE e4 genotype) have also been suggested (Sundstrom et al., 2007). Bushinik et al. observed that 90% of their participants with TBI had abnormalities in at least one pituitary axis (thyroid, adrenal, gonadal axes, and growth hormone function). They found a relationship between lower basal cortisol and higher self-reported fatigue scores (Bushnik et al., 2007). However, a later study by the same group and with a larger sample size did not reproduce these results. No link between neuroendocrine abnormalities and fatigue emerged, but post-TBI fatigue had very robust associations with issues, such as pain, depression, and cognitive problems. They also found that patients taking antidepressant medications reported higher fatigue scores (Englander et al., 2010).

Coping Hypothesis

Because TBI can cause diffuse damage throughout cerebral systems, information processing efficiency and speed are affected. van Zomeren, Brouwer, and Deelman (1984) have suggested the coping hypothesis stipulating that persons with TBI need to use more cerebral resources or need to deploy a greater compensatory mental effort to maintain their levels of performance on daily tasks and activities requiring cognitive resources. This would explain sometimes normal performances on neuropsychological tests followed by a sense of significant fatigue. Indeed, although performance levels may not seem much altered, individuals may deploy increased mental efforts which would result in feelings of tiredness. Such a process seems verifiable since fatigue inducted with tasks in laboratory conditions has been related to certain physiological parameters, such as changes in blood pressure, alterations in white matter integrity, and caudate activation (Riese, Hoedemaeker, Brouwer, & Mulder, 1999; Waljas et al., 2014; Wylie et al., 2017; Wylie & Flashman, 2017; Ziino & Ponsford, 2006). Several studies have revealed a link between post-TBI fatigue and self-reported cognitive distur-bances. This has the potential to significantly impact functioning in daily activities and quality of life (Cantor et al., 2008; Englander et al., 2010; Ouellet & Morin, 2006; Stulemeijer et al., 2008). Although fatigue could contribute to exacerbate cognitive deficits, the inverse relationship could also be true.

Activity Levels and Rest

In a sample of persons having in majority suffered moderate-to-severe TBI who were on average 8 years postinjury, we found that indi-viduals reported an average of 6 naps and 13 rest periods (lying down without sleeping) per week. Despite these very frequent rest periods, the majority of the sample reported feeling significantly fatigued. This led us to conclude that even in the chronic phase several years after moderate-to-severe TBI, rest-seeking behaviors are an important issue which does not seem to be addressed and probably has major impacts on the capacity of these persons to fully engage in their valued roles and activities. In a secondary analysis of this same sample, we observed that persons who reported remaining active through either employ-ment, studying, or engaging in volunteer work were significantly less fatigued than persons who were not active (Ouellet, Morin, & Lavoie, 2009). In a more recent study, we found that work status (i.e., not working) was linked to greater fatigue at 12 months postinjury (Beaulieu-Bonneau & Ouellet, 2016).

Other teams have documented a link between inactivity and fatigue. In a study including patients with moderate-to-severe TBI, Bushnik et al. (2008a) observed that the number of hours they spent being active (e.g., doing housework or school or work-related activities) was inversely correlated with the severity of their fatigue. In a subsequent study, long-term fatigue (persisting beyond 2 years post-TBI) was found to be related to poorer social participation (Lequerica et al., 2017). Taken together, these results suggest a possibly bidirectional relationship between activity (or inactivity) and fatigue. Persons who are less fatigued probably feel more motivated, capable, and disposed to resume work. Conversely, working (or studying) and staying active promote well-being, motivation, pleasure, and satisfaction and thereby decrease fatigue. Furthermore, regular activities, such as work or studying, contribute to a regular routine and schedule. The lack of such a routine may contribute to exacerbate fatigue.

Rest remains a controversial topic after TBI, especially mild TBI. Indeed, although rest might be indicated in the acute phase after a brain injury, in the long term, inactivity linked to rest-seeking is an important problem which probably contributes to perpetuating fatigue and may lead to significant deconditioning (Ouellet & Morin, 2006). In fact, prolonged inactivity is no longer recommended after mild TBI. After a brief initial period rest, it is now recommended that patients swiftly engage into a gradual and controlled return to cognitive activities, nonrisky physical activities and, eventually to normal activities, as tolerated, that is, without a resurgence of symptoms (Giza, Choe, & Barlow, 2018).

Cooccuring Issues: Mood, Disability, Pain, and Sleep Disturbance

Post-TBI fatigue often occurs within a constellation of other symptoms including pain (e.g., headaches), cognitive issues, changes in mood, apathy, loss of motivation or initiative, and disturbed sleep (Beaulieu-Bonneau & Ouellet, 2016; Bushnik et al., 2008b; Cantor et al., 2008; Kempf, Werth, Kaiser, Bassetti, & Baumann, 2010; Lundin, de Boussard, Edman, & Borg, 2006; Meares et al., 2011; Norrie et al., 2010; Ponsford et al., 2012; Stulemeijer et al., 2008). Lequerica et al. examined factors associated with the persistence or remission of fatigue over several years after moderate−severe TBI. They found that persisting fatigue was linked to depression, increased disability, and lingering sleep disturbances (Lequerica et al., 2017). In a longitudinal study of 236 persons with mild-to-severe TBI in the first year postinjury, we found that pain was more clearly linked to post-TBI fatigue early postinjury but not as much later on, perhaps because persons with TBI are more prone to experience pain earlier after the injury (e.g., headaches, injuries to other body areas), or perhaps because people may have adapted to the ongoing presence of pain (Beaulieu-Bonneau & Ouellet, 2016).

Again bidirectional relationships probably exist between fatigue and these cooccurring issues. However, Schonberger et al. examined closely the temporal relation between fatigue, depression, and daytime sleepiness in a cohort of 88 patients with complicated mild–severe TBI. They used a cross-lagged analysis and found that fatigue actually predicted depression and sleepiness, suggesting that fatigue is a primary problem after TBI that probably has a neurological basis and as such should not only be considered as a consequence of other issues, such as depression or sleepiness (Schonberger, Herrberg, & Ponsford, 2014). Post-TBI fatigue thus definitely needs specific attention.

Differentiating Fatigue From Sleepiness

It may be a challenge to distinguish fatigue from excessive daytime sleepiness, especially since the latter is quite common after TBI (Mathias & Alvaro, 2012). In common language, and this includes patients, family members, and health-care providers, there is often a confusion between these problems. One will say "I am tired, I'll go to bed" when in fact the person feels sleepy. However, one can be very fatigued yet not be sleepy, or physiologically ready for sleep. Even some psychometric instruments confuse these constructs by including questions relating both to fatigue and sleepiness. Fatigue refers to a subjective feeling of lassitude, weariness, or depleted energy. The assessment of fatigue is thus mostly subjective (except for measures of specific muscle fatigue). In turn, daytime sleepiness is a physiological state with an increased propensity to fall asleep accompanied by a decrease in alertness (Pigeon, Sateia, & Ferguson, 2003). The person will often present clear signs of sleepiness, such as yawning, eyelids itching, eyelids drooping, and clear decrease in vigilance (e.g., being unable to read, missing parts of a movie).

Evolution of Post–TBI Fatigue and Its Relation to Traumatic Brain Injury Severity

Complaints of fatigue can emerge in the first few days or weeks after TBI (Hutchison, Mainwaring, Comper, Richards, & Bisschop, 2009; Mollayeva et al., 2014; Ouellet & Morin, 2006). Early levels of post-TBI fatigue are an important predictor of fatigue several months later (de Leon et al., 2009; Mollayeva et al., 2014; Norrie et al., 2010; Sundstrom et al., 2007). Unfortunately, fatigue seems to persist for many individuals. It remains as prevalent even several years after the TBI (Olver et al., 1996; Ziino & Ponsford, 2006). Some studies have suggested that fatigue tends to improve over the first year postinjury (Bushnik et al., 2008b), but others have noted a worsening of fatigue (Ponsford & Ziino, 2003; Ponsford et al., 2012; Ziino & Ponsford, 2005). In a systematic review, Mollayeva et al. (2014) pooled prevalence data and found that the mean frequency of significant fatigue tended to decrease slightly with time following the injury, from about 47% at 1 month to 37% at 1 year postinjury. Of note, however, the majority of studies were conducted in samples of persons with mild TBI.

Several studies have not found TBI severity to be a predictor of the prevalence of post-TBI fatigue (Mollayeva et al., 2014; Norrie et al., 2010; Sigurdardottir, Andelic, Roe, & Schanke, 2013). The evolution of post-TBI fatigue may, however, be modulated by TBI severity. The systematic review by Mollayeva et al. (2014) did reveal that fatigue tends to decrease in mild TBI, which is encouraging as the majority of individuals having sustained concussion or mild TBI are expected to no longer experience symptoms by 3−12 months (Carroll et al., 2004; Hall, Hall, & Chapman, 2005).

We found similar results for mild TBI but a different trajectory for more severe injuries. Our team sought to examine more closely the course fatigue over the first year postinjury according to injury severity in a sample of 210 patients. The injury severity composition was 49% mild, 34% moderate, and 18% of severe TBI (Beaulieu-Bonneau & Ouellet, 2016). We used the Multidimensional Fatigue Inventory (MFI) (Smets, Garssen, Bonke, & De Haes, 1995) to document general fatigue, physical fatigue, mental fatigue, and impacts of fatigue on motivation and activity levels. We found that the evolution of fatigue differed according to injury severity: fatigue decreased slightly in the mild TBI subgroup, remained stable in the moderate TBI subgroup, and increased in severe TBI (see Fig. 1.3). Regardless of time since injury, we found that participants with severe TBI displayed higher levels of mental and physical fatigue, as well as reduced activity linked to fatigue. The scores obtained by the whole sample (regardless of TBI severity) were similar to "chronically unwell" individuals assessed in a large-scale validation of the MFI in the US adult population (Lin et al., 2009).

We and other teams thus unfortunately observed that fatigue does not seem to improve over time and may even worsen for persons with moderate or severe TBI (Ponsford & Ziino, 2003; Ponsford et al., 2012; Ziino & Ponsford, 2005). One explanation could lie with issues linked to self-awareness which are much more prominent in more severe injuries, especially early on after the injury. As the patient progresses through rehabilitation and returns gradually to preinjury roles or contexts, this may increase the level of fatigue. In contrast, persons with mild TBI often return quite rapidly to their preinjury activities, thus possibly

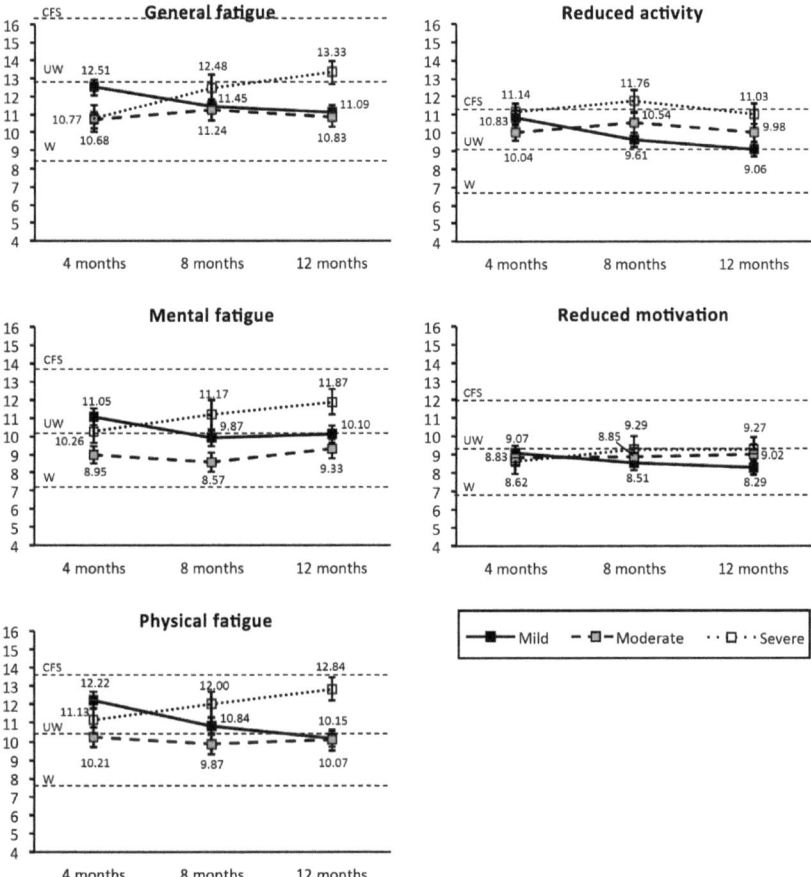

FIGURE 1.3 Results of the MFI subscales over time by severity level. Estimated marginal means with standard errors are given for each subgroup at each assessment (4, 8, 12 months post-TBI). For each MFI subscale, three dotted lines were added, corresponding to the mean scores for three subgroups included in a US adult (aged 18–59) population-based study: CFS-like ($n = 292$), chronically UW ($n = 269$), and W ($n = 222$) (Lin et al., 2009). M ± SD, for CFS, UW, and W subgroups, respectively, are for general fatigue: 16.38 ± 2.73, 12.84 ± 3.93, 8.42 ± 3.59; for mental fatigue: 13.77 ± 3.77, 10.98 ± 4.00, 7.23 ± 3.07; for physical fatigue: 13.63 ± 3.79, 10.39 ± 3.76, 7.77 ± 3.36; for reduced activity: 11.32 ± 4.37, 9.06 ± 3.75, 6.76 ± 2.67; and for reduced motivation: 11.95 ± 3.53, 9.29 ± 3.35, 6.82 ± 2.91. *CFS*, Chronic fatigue syndrome; *MFI*, Multidimensional Fatigue Inventory; *TBI*, traumatic brain injury; *UW*, unwell; *W*, well. *Source: Reproduced with permission from Beaulieu-Bonneau, S., & Ouellet, M. C. (2017). Fatigue in the first year after traumatic brain injury: Course, relationship with injury severity, and correlates. Neuropsychological Rehabilitation, 27(7), 983–1001.*

feeling fatigue earlier on and then gradually adapting or feeling a resolution of their symptoms. Fortunately, there is reason to believe that patients can learn to adapt to the presence of fatigue and to better manage this problem in order to increase their quality of life.

The Phenomenology of Post—TBI Fatigue

Although anyone can relate to the experience of fatigue, the overwhelming and chronic nature of this phenomenon after TBI is known only to those who suffer from it every day. Patients who have participated in our research over the years have provided precious comments which contribute to understanding the experience of post-TBI fatigue (unpublished qualitative data). Many will describe that they have had to learn to identify their own signs of fatigue: for example, they might become impatient (even aggressive), might be irritated by noise, may start making errors or forgetting things, or become unable to keep up with their activities. Activities requiring concentration seem particularly tiring. Several patients also describe that they feel their fatigue coming on rather suddenly, with energy seeming to drop abruptly. Some report "abusing" their energy bank, for example, if they want to finish a task, they will push through but may "pay the price" the next day. Particularly difficult aspects for patients include explaining post-TBI fatigue to others (who might interpret fatigue as a lack of motivation) and most importantly, accepting that fatigue is present daily, does not seem to go away, and realizing how it limits activities. Interestingly, comments also emerge about gradually learning to adapt to fatigue: some will say that with time, one can learn to adapt to fatigue and to be aware of one's energy level, and thus compose with it. Understanding one's own difficulties is key, it allows one to recover confidence and organize life and activities more efficiently. Some use a battery metaphor, reporting that they need to stay aware of their "battery level" throughout the day so as not to empty it too quickly because it does not recharge as effectively as before. Taking regular breaks allows them to avoid errors and falling into the "red zone." Specific strategies include naps, listening to music, and exercising.

Theadom et al. (2016) qualitatively investigated the experience of fatigue and sleep over the first 2 years after mild-to-severe TBI in 30 participants. The longitudinal design allowed the documentation of an evolution and variability of attitudes and experiences about fatigue over time. Four main themes were found: (1) making sense of fatigue and sleep, (2) accepting the need to rest, (3) learning how to rest, and (4) the impacts of needing to rest on life activities. Although it presents realities long known to rehabilitation professionals working with TBI patients in the chronic phase, this study is particularly informative on the long-term adaptation to fatigue from the patient's point of view.

First, participants expressed that they had to go through a process of making sense of their fatigue. The authors found that at 6 months post-injury, persons with TBI were only just starting to apprehend the chronic reality of their fatigue. Of note, participants reported that they did not feel prepared for the intensity and persistence of fatigue. In this sense the present manual may help support the process of becoming aware of the impacts of fatigue and learning to adapt to this new symptom. For example, filling out a self-monitoring tool, such as an energy/activity diary, allows the patient to take note of needs for rest during different times of day, linking other health habits with fatigue, for example, sleep, exercise or eating habits, and evaluating how differ-ent activities may need to be adapted to take into account present limitations.

A second theme identified by Theadom et al. was "Accepting the need for rest." At 6 months postinjury, many participants reported that they tended to push themselves too much, describing that they then reached a point where they need to stop completely and rest, a phenomenon referred to as the "Boom and Bust cycle" in some litera-tures relative to chronic fatigue or illness-related fatigue. This overexer-tion phenomenon also seemed to be associated with feelings of guilt about not being able to complete activities as wished or as compared to before the accident. The notion of acceptance here suggests that the pro-cess may imply significant frustration for many patients, as they come to realize and accept that they need either to rest or to adjust their activ-ities to manage their new "energy bank."

Treatment Options for Fatigue

Although fatigue is recognized in clinical settings, it remains unclear how fatigue is monitored and managed, and scientific efforts toward the understanding of the issue of fatigue after TBI have been at best timid until now. No particular medication has emerged as an effective agent to treat post-TBI fatigue. Behavioral strategies, and adaptations of the environment thus represent important management venues but have not been well documented in the literature.

Pharmacological Treatment

No medication has emerged as an effective treatment for post-TBI fatigue. There have been anecdotal reports of some success in neurological patients (not necessarily TBI) with amantadine, methylphe-nidate, bromocriptine, pemoline, phenylephrine, and amphetamines

(Chaudhuri & Behan, 2004; Elovic, Dobrovic, & Fellus, 2005). Modafinil, which is mostly used in the context of narcolepsy, has received the most scientific attention. A study by Jha et al. did not find modafinil to be more beneficial than a placebo and the authors concluded that post-TBI fatigue is a complex and multifactorial phenomenon, and that its treatment necessitates a multifaceted approach (Jha et al., 2008). Some authors have suggested that the affective components of fatigue (depression, anxiety) may respond to antidepressant or anxiolytic medications, particularly the more energizing antidepressants, such as certain SSRIs (Chaudhuri & Behan, 2004; De Groot, Phillips, & Eskes, 2003) but these effects and the safety of these in this context have not been studied adequately.

Exercise

Physical activity is known to improve symptoms of fatigue in various medical conditions including chronic fatigue syndrome (CFS) (Hilfiker et al., 2018; Kelley & Kelley, 2017; Wessely, David, Butler, & Chalder, 1989), but the evidence for TBI per se is still quite limited (Larun, Brurberg, Odgaard-Jensen, & Price, 2017; Xu, Li, Wang, & Cao, 2017). Driver and Ede (2009) observed that an 8-week program of aquatic exercises (three sessions per week) led to improvements in anxiety, depression, anger, confusion as well as a reduction in fatigue and an increase in vigor after TBI. Another team evaluated the efficacy of a home-based walking intervention over a 12-week period. The intervention involved a pedometer to increase walking, and calls were made to participants by coaches. A control condition used nutritional counseling. Significant decreases were observed on several measures of fatigue and the improvements seemed to be well maintained at a 12-week follow-up (Kolakowsky-Hayner et al., 2017). These results are encouraging and suggest that a low-cost and accessible option, such as walking, can have benefits on post-TBI fatigue while improving other health parameters. Although the challenges of increasing physical exercise are well known, walking may be a good way to start motivating some patients to increase physical activity levels.

Education About Health-Related Habits and the Environment

Education about sleep hygiene is often suggested, as well as the effects of ingesting products with stimulant effects (e.g., smoking, energy drinks, chocolate, ginseng, *Ginkgo biloba*). Indeed, although some products may seem to have some short-term benefits to manage fatigue, their timing and dosage may have direct detrimental on nighttime sleep quality and can contribute to stress or anxiety.

Light Therapy

In the first randomized trial of light therapy for fatigue after TBI, Sinclair et al. (2014) observed a significant reduction in fatigue in persons who were administered 4 weeks of short wavelength blue light therapy (45 min/day at home) compared to a placebo yellow light. This is a promising treatment option which could be offered in complement to cognitive and behavioral interventions.

Cognitive and Behavioral Strategies

A variety of behavioral strategies have been proposed to manage fatigue secondary to neurological disorders, for example, interventions to reduce stress, pacing, rescheduling activities at times when energy is the highest, changing the environment, and delegating chores (De Groot et al., 2003; Ward & Winters, 2003).

Since research on the management of post-TBI fatigue is only at its infancy, we can look to research and practice in other populations, for example, multiple sclerosis or CFS. Research in the field of CFS has shown that individuals will often limit their physical activity levels. This decrease in activity is also observed in other dimensions of life, for example, in terms of social or leisure activities. Patients may believe that engaging in activities will worsen their situation. They can also have recurrent thoughts about needing to rest. In the CFS literature, cognitive–behavioral interventions thus typically include a gradual increase in activity levels (Driver & Ede, 2009; Gordon et al., 1998; Price, Mitchell, Tidy, & Hunot, 2008; Vos-Vromans et al., 2012).

The National Institute for Clinical Excellence in the United Kingdom (NICE, 2007) is quite clear relative to the management of CFS or myalgic encephalomyelitis: specialized care should be offered and this mainly involves cognitive and behavioral interventions, such as pacing, activity management, CBT, graded exercise, and management of cooccurring physical and emotional symptoms. The goal of these interventions should be to maintain or gradually improve physical, emotional, and cognitive capacities.

More specifically, the NICE guidelines suggest that CBT should ideally be administered individually using a collaborative approach (shared formulation, agreement on therapeutic goals, and tailoring the intervention to the patient's needs, preferences, and characteristics). Psychoeducation should be included, for example, explaining the relationship between symptoms and thoughts, feelings, behaviors, and helping the patient to identify causal and perpetuating factors. The guideline clearly recommends the use of self-monitoring of patterns of activity, rest, thoughts, feelings, and behaviors. Cognitive therapy components are suggested, such as developing awareness of thoughts and attitudes, challenging dysfunctional fatigue-related thoughts and behaviors. Attention to hypervigilance and reassurance-seeking behaviors is also underscored and refocusing/distraction techniques are suggested. Behavioral experiments are also proposed to test alternative behaviors, thoughts, or beliefs, including pleasurable and satisfying activities (which foster a sense of mastery and accomplishment). Other strategies may include building problem-solving, assertion or communication skills, and behavioral strategies to improve sleep and stress management techniques (e.g., breathing, relaxation training). Preparing the person for long-term maintenance of improvements and strategies to manage setbacks or relapses are also important (NICE, 2007).

Research on the efficacy of CBT specifically for fatigue only in the context of TBI is still lacking. However, a few studies (from our group as well as others) have incorporated fatigue management with cognitive–behavioral interventions for insomnia (Nguyen et al., 2019; Ouellet & Morin, 2004, 2007) with some success translating in reductions on self-reported fatigue scales. In their randomized controlled trial for insomnia and fatigue in TBI and stroke patients, Nguyen et al. (2019) included therapeutic components which they described as reorganizing daily schedules (pacing of tasks, breaks, improving sleep hygiene), graded activity, and strategies for managing physical and mental fatigue (environmental modifications, management of time pressure). Their results are very encouraging as daily fatigue levels were significantly reduced with this intervention.

In our own work the fatigue management module we have developed (and incorporated into the CBT for insomnia protocol) included the following: completing an energy activity daily diary describing information about activities and levels of fatigue at different times of the day, learning to identify signs of one's own of fatigue, determining patterns of energy relative to activities (e.g., identifying optimal periods of energy, spotting occurrence of "boom and bust" behavior), discussing priorities, responsibilities, and avoidance of activities, contemplating the integration or reintegration of some activities which could provide pleasure, mastery and energy, realistic planning of activities, providing strategies to pace of activities (alternating between different types of activities, separating tasks into manageable units, and incorporation of breaks). We also explored thoughts, attitudes, and beliefs about fatigue and alternative ways to rest. The person was encouraged to gradually augment levels of activity, not only physical but also in the social and leisure spheres.

INTERACTION BETWEEN INSOMNIA AND FATIGUE

Our research has shown that insomnia and fatigue are two independent phenomena that influence each other. Indeed, among persons who did not have any symptoms of insomnia after TBI, we still found that 60% reported suffering from significant fatigue. For those who did suffer from insomnia, 86% also suffered from clinically significant fatigue. Insomnia can most certainly bring its own share of fatigue either by exacerbating the fatigue already caused by TBI, or by creating an independent tiredness, solely related to having sleep difficulties (Ouellet et al., 2006; Ouellet & Morin, 2006).

Of note, our treatment studies showed that despite improving sleep quality, CBT did not completely alleviate fatigue, suggesting that a good part of the fatigue is independent of sleep difficulties after TBI. Indeed, the improvements in nocturnal sleep were accompanied by decreases in general fatigue or physical fatigue, but not in mental fatigue which is a very common persisting complaint following TBI. These mitigated results possibly can be explained by the fact that we incorporated fatigue strategies only in the last four sessions of treatment. Some patients may benefit from a full course of treatment specifically focused on fatigue over several weeks or months. Unfortunately, research is not advanced enough to suggest any particular intensity or duration of treatment. However, Theadom's qualitative research (Theadom et al., 2016) described earlier is quite eloquent by showing that the processes of developing awareness and eventually adapting to fatigue probably take months, perhaps years, for some patients. As such, the CBT treatment proposed in this manual should be adapted to individual needs of patients. Whereas a course of 8 weeks of CBT is known to improve insomnia after TBI, the strategies for fatigue probably need to be implemented on a longer period. We hope this manual will stimulate further research relative to these two very important persisting sequelae of TBI.

References

Allain, P., Togher, L., & Azouvi, P. (2018). Social cognition and traumatic brain injury: Current knowledge. *Brain Injury*, 1−3. Available from https://doi.org/10.1080/02699052.2018.1533143.

Alway, Y., Gould, K. R., Johnston, L., McKenzie, D., & Ponsford, J. (2016). A prospective examination of Axis I psychiatric disorders in the first 5 years following moderate to severe traumatic brain injury. *Psychological Medicine*, 46(6), 1331−1341. Available from https://doi.org/10.1017/S0033291715002986. Retrieved from <https://www.ncbi.nlm.nih.gov/pubmed/26867715>.

American Academy of Sleep Medicine. (2014). *International classification of sleep disorders: Diagnostic and coding manual, 3rd ed (ICSD-3)*. Westchester, IL: American Academy of Sleep Medicine.

American Psychiatric Association. (2013). *Diagnostic and statistical manual of mental disorders, 5th edition (DSM-5)*. Washington, DC: American Psychiatric Publishing.

Andelic, N., Howe, E. I., Hellstrom, T., Sanchez, M. F., Lu, J., Lovstad, M., & Roe, C. (2018). Disability and quality of life 20 years after traumatic brain injury. *Brain and Behavior*, 8(7), e01018. Available from https://doi.org/10.1002/brb3.1018.

Ao, K. H., Ho, C. H., Wang, C. C., Wang, J. J., Chio, C. C., & Kuo, J. R. (2017). The increased risk of stroke in early insomnia following traumatic brain injury: A population-based cohort study. *Sleep Medicine*, 37, 187−192. Available from https://doi.org/10.1016/j.sleep.2017.02.010.

Ashman, T. A., Cantor, J. B., Gordon, W. A., Spielman, L., Egan, M., Ginsberg, A., ... Flanagan, S. (2008). Objective measurement of fatigue following traumatic brain injury. *Journal of Head Trauma Rehabilitation*, 23(1), 33−40. Available from https://doi.org/10.1097/01.HTR.0000308719.70288.22. Retrieved from <http://www.ncbi.nlm.nih.gov/entrez/query.fcgi?cmd = Retrieve&db = PubMed&dopt = Citation&list_uids = 18219233>.

Ballesio, A., Aquino, M., Feige, B., Johann, A. F., Kyle, S. D., Spiegelhalder, K., ... Baglioni, C. (2018). The effectiveness of behavioural and cognitive behavioural therapies for insomnia on depressive and fatigue symptoms: A systematic review and network meta-analysis. *Sleep Medicine Reviews*, 37, 114−129. Available from https://doi.org/10.1016/j.smrv.2017.01.006.

Barker-Collo, S., Jones, K., Theadom, A., Starkey, N., Dowell, A., McPherson, K., ... Feigin, V. (2015). Neuropsychological outcome and its correlates in the first year after adult mild traumatic brain injury: A population-based New Zealand study. *Brain Injury*, 29 (13−14), 1604−1616. Available from https://doi.org/10.3109/02699052.2015.1075143.

Baumann, C. R., Bassetti, C. L., Valko, P. O., Haybaeck, J., Keller, M., Clark, E., ... Scammell, T. E. (2009). Loss of hypocretin (orexin) neurons with traumatic brain injury. *Annals of Neurology*, 66(4), 555−559. Available from https://doi.org/10.1002/ana.21836. Retrieved from <http://www.ncbi.nlm.nih.gov/entrez/query.fcgi?cmd = Retrieve&db = PubMed&dopt = Citation&list_uids = 19847903>.

Baumann, C. R., Stocker, R., Imhof, H. G., Trentz, O., Hersberger, M., Mignot, E., & Bassetti, C. L. (2005). Hypocretin-1 (orexin A) deficiency in acute traumatic brain injury. *Neurology*, 65(1), 147−149. Available from https://doi.org/10.1212/01.wnl.0000167605.02541.f2. Retrieved from <http://www.ncbi.nlm.nih.gov/entrez/query.fcgi?cmd = Retrieve&db = PubMed&dopt = Citation&list_uids = 16009905>.

Baumann, C. R., Werth, E., Stocker, R., Ludwig, S., & Bassetti, C. L. (2007). Sleep-wake disturbances 6 months after traumatic brain injury: A prospective study. *Brain*, 130(Pt 7), 1873−1883. Available from https://doi.org/10.1093/brain/awm109. Retrieved from <http://www.ncbi.nlm.nih.gov/entrez/query.fcgi?cmd = Retrieve&db = PubMed&dopt = Citation&list_uids = 17584779>.

Bayen, E., Pradat-Diehl, P., Jourdan, C., Ghout, I., Bosserelle, V., Azerad, S., ... Steering Committee of the Pari, S. T. B. I. s. (2013). Predictors of informal care burden 1 year after a severe traumatic brain injury: Results from the PariS-TBI study. *Journal of Head Trauma Rehabilitation*, 28(6), 408−418. Available from https://doi.org/10.1097/HTR.0b013e31825413cf. Retrieved from <http://www.ncbi.nlm.nih.gov/pubmed/22691963>.

Beaulieu-Bonneau, S., & Ouellet, M. C. (2016). Fatigue in the first year after traumatic brain injury: Course, relationship with injury severity, and correlates. *Neuropsychological Rehabilitation*, 27, 983−1001.

Beetar, J. T., Guilmette, T. J., & Sparadeo, F. R. (1996). Sleep and pain complaints in symptomatic traumatic brain injury and neurologic populations. *Archives of Physical Medicine and Rehabilitation*, 77(12), 1298−1302. Available from https://doi.org/10.1016/S0003-9993(96)90196-3. Retrieved from <http://www.ncbi.nlm.nih.gov/entrez/query.fcgi?cmd = Retrieve&db = PubMed&dopt = Citation&list_uids = 8976315>.

Belmont, A., Agar, N., Hugeron, C., Gallais, B., & Azouvi, P. (2006a). Fatigue and traumatic brain injury. *Annales de Réadaptation et de Médecine Physique*, 49(6), 370−384. Retrieved from <http://www.ncbi.nlm.nih.gov/entrez/query.fcgi?cmd = Retrieve&db = PubMed&dopt = Citation&list_uids = 16716438>.

Belmont, A., Agar, N., Hugeron, C., Gallais, B., & Azouvi, P. (2006b). Fatigue and traumatic brain injury. *Annales de Réadaptation et de Médecine Physique*, 49(6), 283−288.

Available from https://doi.org/10.1016/j.annrmp.2006.04.017. 370−374. Retrieved from <http://www.ncbi.nlm.nih.gov/pubmed/16716438>.

Bier, N., Dutil, E., & Couture, M. (2009). Factors affecting leisure participation after a traumatic brain injury: An exploratory study. *Journal of Head Trauma Rehabilitation, 24*(3), 187−194. Available from https://doi.org/10.1097/HTR.0b013e3181a0b15a.

Billiard, M., & Podesta, C. (2013). Recurrent hypersomnia following traumatic brain injury. *Sleep Medicine, 14*(5), 462−465. Available from https://doi.org/10.1016/j.sleep.2013.01.009.

Blais, M.-C., & Boivert, J.-M. (2005). Psychological and marital adjustment in couples following a traumatic brain injury (TBI): A critical review. *Brain Injury, 19*(14), 1223−1235.

Boake, C., McCauley, S. R., Levin, H. S., Pedroza, C., Contant, C. F., Song, J. X., ... Diaz-Marchan, P. J. (2005). Diagnostic criteria for postconcussional syndrome after mild to moderate traumatic brain injury. *The Journal of Neuropsychiatry and Clinical Neurosciences, 17*(3), 350−356. Available from https://doi.org/10.1176/jnp.17.3.350.

Bombardier, C. H., Hoekstra, T., Dikmen, S., & Fann, J. R. (2016). Depression trajectories during the first year after traumatic brain injury. *Journal of Neurotrauma.* Available from https://doi.org/10.1089/neu.2015.4349.

Bootzin, R. R., Epstein, D., & Wood, J. M. (1991). Stimulus control instructions. In P. J. Hauri (Ed.), *Case studies in insomnia* (pp. 19−28). New York: Plenum.

Bruns, J., Jr., & Hauser, W. A. (2003). The epidemiology of traumatic brain injury: A review. *Epilepsia., 44*(Suppl 10), 2−10.

Bryant, R. A., O'Donnell, M. L., Creamer, M., McFarlane, A. C., Clark, C. R., & Silove, D. (2010). The psychiatric sequelae of traumatic injury. *American Journal of Psychiatry, 167* (3), 312−320. Available from https://doi.org/10.1176/appi.ajp.2009.09050617, Retrieved from <Go to ISI>://WOS:000275056300013.

Bushnik, T., Englander, J., & Katznelson, L. (2007). Fatigue after TBI: Association with neuroendocrine abnormalities. *Brain Injury, 21*(6), 559−566. Available from https://doi.org/10.1080/02699050701426915. Retrieved from <http://www.ncbi.nlm.nih.gov/entrez/query.fcgi?cmd = Retrieve&db = PubMed&dopt = Citation&list_uids = 17577706>.

Bushnik, T., Englander, J., & Wright, J. (2008a). The experience of fatigue in the first 2 years after moderate-to-severe traumatic brain injury: A preliminary report. *Journal of Head Trauma Rehabilitation, 23*(1), 17−24. Available from https://doi.org/10.1097/01.HTR.0000308717.80590.22. Retrieved from <http://www.ncbi.nlm.nih.gov/entrez/query.fcgi?cmd = Retrieve&db = PubMed&dopt = Citation&list_uids = 18219231>. 00001199-200801000-00005 [pii].

Bushnik, T., Englander, J., & Wright, J. (2008b). Patterns of fatigue and its correlates over the first 2 years after traumatic brain injury. *Journal of Head Trauma Rehabilitation, 23*(1), 25−32. Available from https://doi.org/10.1097/01.HTR.0000308718.88214.bb. Retrieved from <http://www.ncbi.nlm.nih.gov/entrez/query.fcgi?cmd = Retrieve&db = PubMed&dopt = Citation&list_uids = 18219232>.

Cantor, J. B., Ashman, T., Gordon, W., Ginsberg, A., Engmann, C., Egan, M., ... Flanagan, S. (2008). Fatigue after traumatic brain injury and its impact on participation and quality of life. *Journal of Head Trauma Rehabilitation, 23*(1), 41−51. Available from https://doi.org/10.1097/01.HTR.0000308720.70288.af. Retrieved from <http://www.ncbi.nlm.nih.gov/entrez/query.fcgi?cmd = Retrieve&db = PubMed&dopt = Citation&list_uids = 18219234>.

Cantor, J. B., Bushnik, T., Cicerone, K., Dijkers, M. P., Gordon, W., Hammond, F. M., ... Spielman, L. A. (2012). Insomnia, fatigue, and sleepiness in the first 2 years after traumatic brain injury: An NIDRR TBI model system module study. *Journal of Head Trauma Rehabilitation, 27*(6), E1−14. Available from https://doi.org/10.1097/HTR.0b013e318270f91e.

Cantor, J. B., Gordon, W., & Gumber, S. (2013). What is post TBI fatigue? *NeuroRehabilitation, 32*(4), 875−883. Available from https://doi.org/10.3233/NRE-130912. Retrieved from <http://www.ncbi.nlm.nih.gov/pubmed/23867414>.

Carlozzi, N. E., Kratz, A. L., Sander, A. M., Chiaravalloti, N. D., Brickell, T. A., Lange, R. T., ... Tulsky, D. S. (2015). Health-related quality of life in caregivers of individuals with traumatic brain injury: Development of a conceptual model. *Archives of Physical Medicine and Rehabilitation, 96*(1), 105–113. Available from https://doi.org/10.1016/j.apmr.2014.08.021. Retrieved from <http://www.ncbi.nlm.nih.gov/pubmed/25239281>.

Carroll, L. J., Cassidy, J. D., Cancelliere, C., Cote, P., Hincapie, C. A., Kristman, V. L., ... Hartvigsen, J. (2014). Systematic review of the prognosis after mild traumatic brain injury in adults: Cognitive, psychiatric, and mortality outcomes: Results of the International Collaboration on Mild Traumatic Brain Injury Prognosis. *Archives of Physical Medicine and Rehabilitation, 95*(3 Suppl.), S152–173. Available from https://doi.org/10.1016/j.apmr.2013.08.300.

Carroll, L. J., Cassidy, J. D., Peloso, P. M., Borg, J., von Holst, H., Holm, L., ... Pepin, M. (2004). Prognosis for mild traumatic brain injury: Results of the WHO Collaborating Centre Task Force on Mild Traumatic Brain Injury. *Journal of Rehabilitation Medicine, 43 Suppl.*, 84–105. Retrieved from <http://www.ncbi.nlm.nih.gov/entrez/query.fcgi?cmd = Retrieve&db = PubMed&dopt = Citation&list_uids = 15083873>.

Castriotta, R. J., Wilde, M. C., Lai, J. M., Atanasov, S., Masel, B. E., & Kuna, S. T. (2007). Prevalence and consequences of sleep disorders in traumatic brain injury. *Journal of Clinical Sleep Medicine, 3*(4), 349–356.

Cassidy, J. D., Carroll, L. J., Peloso, P. M., Borg, J., von Holst, H., Holm, L., ... Injury, W. H. O. C. C. T. F. o. M. T. B. (2004). Incidence, risk factors and prevention of mild traumatic brain injury: results of the WHO Collaborating Centre Task Force on Mild Traumatic Brain Injury. *J Rehabil Med* (43 Suppl), 28–60, Retrieved from. Available from http://www.ncbi.nlm.nih.gov/pubmed/15083870.

Chaput, G., Giguere, J. F., Chauny, J. M., Denis, R., & Lavigne, G. (2009). Relationship among subjective sleep complaints, headaches, and mood alterations following a mild traumatic brain injury. *Sleep Medicine, 10*(7), 713–716. Available from https://doi.org/10.1016/j.sleep.2008.07.015. Retrieved from <http://www.ncbi.nlm.nih.gov/pubmed/19147402>.

Chaudhuri, A., & Behan, P. O. (2004). Fatigue in neurological disorders. *Lancet, 363*(9413), 978–988. Retrieved from <http://www.ncbi.nlm.nih.gov/entrez/query.fcgi?cmd = Retrieve&db = PubMed&dopt = Citation&list_uids = 15043967>.

Chin, L. M., Keyser, R. E., Dsurney, J., & Chan, L. (2015). Improved cognitive performance following aerobic exercise training in people with traumatic brain injury. *Archives of Physical Medicine and Rehabilitation, 96*(4), 754–759. Available from https://doi.org/10.1016/j.apmr.2014.11.009.

Chiu, H. Y., Chen, P. Y., Chen, N. H., Chuang, L. P., & Tsai, P. S. (2013). Trajectories of sleep changes during the acute phase of traumatic brain injury: A 7-day actigraphy study. *Journal of the Formosan Medical Association, 112*(9), 545–553. Available from https://doi.org/10.1016/j.jfma.2013.06.007.

Chiu, H. Y., Lin, E. Y., Wei, L., Lin, J. H., Lee, H. C., Fan, Y. C., & Tsai, P. S. (2015). Hypnotics use but not insomnia increased the risk of dementia in traumatic brain injury patients. *European Neuropsychopharmacology, 25*(12), 2271–2277. Available from https://doi.org/10.1016/j.euroneuro.2015.09.011.

Cicerone, K. D., & Maestas, K. L. (2014). *Rehabilitation of attention and executive function impairments. Handbook on the neuropsychology of traumatic brain injury* (pp. 191–211). Springer.

Cohen, M., Oksenberg, A., Snir, D., Stern, M. J., & Groswasser, Z. (1992). Temporally related changes of sleep complaints in traumatic brain injured patients. *Journal of Neurology, Neurosurgery, and Psychiatry, 55*(4), 313–315. Retrieved from <http://www.ncbi.nlm.nih.gov/entrez/query.fcgi?cmd = Retrieve&db = PubMed&dopt = Citation&list_uids = 1583518>.

Corrigan, J. D., & Hammond, F. M. (2013). Traumatic brain injury as a chronic health condition. *Archives of Physical Medicine and Rehabilitation, 94*(6), 1199–1201. Available from https://doi.org/10.1016/j.apmr.2013.01.023.

Cullen, N., Meyer, M. J., Aubut, J. -A., Bayley, M., & Teasell, R. (2013). *Evidence-based review of moderate to severe acquired brain injury: Module 3—Efficacy and models of care following acquired brain injury.* In ABIEBR (Ed.). Retrieved from <www.abiebr.com>.

Dahm, J., & Ponsford, J. (2015a). Comparison of long-term outcomes following traumatic injury: What is the unique experience for those with brain injury compared with orthopaedic injury? *Injury, 46*(1), 142–149. Available from https://doi.org/10.1016/j.injury.2014.07.012.

Dahm, J., & Ponsford, J. (2015b). Long-term employment outcomes following traumatic brain injury and orthopaedic trauma: A ten-year prospective study. *Journal of Rehabilitation Medicine, 47*(10), 932–940. Available from https://doi.org/10.2340/16501977-2016.

Dahm, J., & Ponsford, J. (2015c). Predictors of global functioning and employment 10 years following traumatic brain injury compared with orthopaedic injury. *Brain Injury, 29* (13–14), 1539–1546. Available from https://doi.org/10.3109/02699052.2015.1075141. Retrieved from <http://www.ncbi.nlm.nih.gov/pubmed/26379124>.

Damiano, D. L., Zampieri, C., Ge, J., Acevedo, A., & Dsurney, J. (2016). Effects of a rapid-resisted elliptical training program on motor, cognitive and neurobehavioral functioning in adults with chronic traumatic brain injury. *Experimental Brain Research, 234*(8), 2245–2252. Available from https://doi.org/10.1007/s00221-016-4630-8.

De Groot, M. H., Phillips, S. J., & Eskes, G. A. (2003). Fatigue associated with stroke and other neurologic conditions: Implications for stroke rehabilitation. *Archives of Physical Medicine and Rehabilitation, 84*(11), 1714–1720. Retrieved from <http://www.ncbi.nlm.nih.gov/entrez/query.fcgi?cmd = Retrieve&db = PubMed&dopt = Citation&list_uids = 14639575>. doi:S0003999303003460 [pii].

De La Rue-Evans, L., Nesbitt, K., & Oka, R. K. (2013). Sleep hygiene program implementation in patients with traumatic brain injury. *Rehabilitation Nursing, 38*(1), 2–10. Available from https://doi.org/10.1002/rnj.1066.

de Leon, M. B., Kirsch, N. L., Maio, R. F., Tan-Schriner, C. U., Millis, S. R., Frederiksen, S., ... Breer, M. L. (2009). Baseline predictors of fatigue 1 year after mild head injury. *Archives of Physical Medicine and Rehabilitation, 90*(6), 956–965. Available from https://doi.org/10.1016/j.apmr.2008.12.016. Retrieved from <http://www.ncbi.nlm.nih.gov/pubmed/19480871>.

Degeneffe, C. E. (2001). Family caregiving and traumatic brain injury. *Health & Social Work, 26*(4), 257–268. Retrieved from <http://www.ncbi.nlm.nih.gov/pubmed/11758867>.

Demakis, G. J., Hammond, F. M., & Knotts, A. (2010). Prediction of depression and anxiety 1 year after moderate-severe traumatic brain injury. *Applied Neuropsychology, 17*(3), 183–189. Available from https://doi.org/10.1080/09084282.2010.499752. Retrieved from <http://www.ncbi.nlm.nih.gov/pubmed/20799109>.

Diaz, A. P., Schwarzbold, M. L., Thais, M. E., Hohl, A., Bertotti, M. M., Schmoeller, R., ... Guarnieri, R. (2012). Psychiatric disorders and health-related quality of life after severe traumatic brain injury: A prospective study. *Journal of Neurotrauma, 29*(6), 1029–1037.

Doyle, S. T., Perrin, P. B., Diaz Sosa, D. M., Espinosa Jove, I. G., Lee, G. K., & Arango-Lasprilla, J. C. (2013). Connecting family needs and TBI caregiver mental health in Mexico City, Mexico. *Brain Injury, 27*(12), 1441–1449. Available from https://doi.org/10.3109/02699052.2013.826505. Retrieved from <http://www.ncbi.nlm.nih.gov/pubmed/23957747>.

Driver, S., & Ede, A. (2009). Impact of physical activity on mood after TBI. *Brain Injury, 23* (3), 203–212. Available from https://doi.org/10.1080/02699050802695574. Retrieved from <http://www.ncbi.nlm.nih.gov/entrez/query.fcgi?cmd = Retrieve&db = PubMed &dopt = Citation&list_uids = 19205956>. 908612884 [pii].

Duclos, C., Dumont, M., Arbour, C., Paquet, J., Blais, H., Menon, D. K., ... Gosselin, N. (2017). Parallel recovery of consciousness and sleep in acute traumatic brain injury. *Neurology, 88*(3), 268−275.

Duclos, C., Dumont, M., Blais, H., Paquet, J., Laflamme, E., de Beaumont, L., ... Gosselin, N. (2013). Rest-activity cycle disturbances in the acute phase of moderate to severe traumatic brain injury. *Neurorehabilitation and Neural Repair.* Available from https://doi.org/10.1177/1545968313517756.

Duclos, C., Dumont, M., Potvin, M. J., Desautels, A., Gilbert, D., Menon, D. K., ... Gosselin, N. (2016). Evolution of severe sleep-wake cycle disturbances following traumatic brain injury: A case study in both acute and subacute phases post-injury. *BMC Neurology, 16*(1), 186. Available from https://doi.org/10.1212/wnl.0000000000003508.

Edinger, J. D., & Carney, C. E. (2008). *Overcoming insomnia: A cognitive-behavioral therapy approach, therapist guide.* New York: Oxford University Press.

Elovic, E. P., Dobrovic, N. M., & Fellus, J. L. (2005). Fatigue after traumatic brain injury. In J. DeLuca (Ed.), *Fatigue as a window to the brain* (pp. 89−106). Cambridge, MA: Massachusetts Institute of Technology.

Englander, J., Bushnik, T., Oggins, J., & Katznelson, L. (2010). Fatigue after traumatic brain injury: Association with neuroendocrine, sleep, depression and other factors. *Brain Injury, 24*(12), 1379−1388. Available from https://doi.org/10.3109/02699052.2010.523041. Retrieved from <http://www.ncbi.nlm.nih.gov/pubmed/20961172>.

Esbjornsson, E., Skoglund, T., & Sunnerhagen, K. S. (2013). Fatigue, psychosocial adaptation and quality of life one year after traumatic brain injury and suspected traumatic axonal injury; evaluations of patients and relatives: A pilot study. *Journal of Rehabilitation Medicine, 45*(8), 771−777. Available from https://doi.org/10.2340/16501977-1170. Retrieved from <http://www.ncbi.nlm.nih.gov/pubmed/24002313>.

Eslinger, P. J., Zappala, G., Chakara, F., & Barrett, A. M. (2012). Cognitive Impairments. In N. D. Zasler, D. I. Katz, & R. Z. Zafonte (Eds.), *Brain Injury Medicine* (2nd Edition, pp. 990−1001). New York: Demos Medical Publishing.

Espie, C. A. (2002). Insomnia: Conceptual issues in the development, persistence, and treatment of sleep disorder in adults. *Annual Review of Psychology, 53*, 215−243. Available from https://doi.org/10.1146/annurev.psych.53.100901.135243. Retrieved from <http://www.ncbi.nlm.nih.gov/entrez/query.fcgi?cmd = Retrieve&db = PubMed &dopt = Citation&list_uids = 11752485>.

Fakhran, S., Yaeger, K., & Alhilali, L. (2013). Symptomatic white matter changes in mild traumatic brain injury resemble pathologic features of early Alzheimer dementia. *Radiology, 269*(1), 249−257. Available from https://doi.org/10.1148/radiol.13122343.

Farrell-Carnahan, L., Barnett, S., Lamberty, G., Hammond, F. M., Kretzmer, T. S., Franke, L. M., ... Nakase-Richardson, R. (2015). Insomnia symptoms and behavioural health symptoms in veterans 1 year after traumatic brain injury. *Brain Injury, 1−9.* Retrieved from <https://www.ncbi.nlm.nih.gov/pubmed/26274494>.

Faul, M., Xu, L., Wald, M. M., & Coronado, V. G. (2010). *Traumatic brain injury in the United States: Emergency department visits, hospitalizations and deaths 2002-2006.* Atlanta, GA: National Center for Injury Prevention and Control, Centers for Disease Control and Prevention. Retrieved from <http://www.cdc.gov/traumaticbraininjury/pdf/blue_book.pdf>.

Ferguson, J. M. (2001). SSRI antidepressant medications: Adverse effects and tolerability. *Primary Care Companion to the Journal of Clinical Psychiatry, 3*(1), 22−27. Retrieved from <http://www.ncbi.nlm.nih.gov/entrez/query.fcgi?cmd = Retrieve&db = PubMed &dopt = Citation&list_uids = 15014625>.

Fichtenberg, N. L., Millis, S. R., Mann, N. R., Zafonte, R. D., & Millard, A. E. (2000). Factors associated with insomnia among post-acute traumatic brain injury survivors. *Brain Injury, 14*(7), 659−667. Retrieved from <http://www.ncbi.nlm.nih.gov/entrez/query.fcgi?cmd = Retrieve&db = PubMed&dopt = Citation&list_uids = 10914647>.

Flanagan, S. R., Greenwald, B., & Wieber, S. (2007). Pharmacological treatment of insomnia for individuals with brain injury. *Journal of Head Trauma Rehabilitation, 22*(1), 67–70. Retrieved from <http://www.ncbi.nlm.nih.gov/entrez/query.fcgi?cmd = Retrieve&db = PubMed&dopt = Citation&list_uids = 17235234>. doi:00001199-200701000-00009 [pii].

Fogelberg, D. J., Hoffman, J. M., Dikmen, S., Temkin, N. R., & Bell, K. R. (2012). Association of sleep and co-occurring psychological conditions at 1 year after traumatic brain injury. *Archives of Physical Medicine and Rehabilitation, 93*(8), 1313–1318. Available from https://doi.org/10.1016/j.apmr.2012.04.031. Retrieved from <http://www.ncbi.nlm.nih.gov/pubmed/22840828>.

Friese, R. S., Diaz-Arrastia, R., McBride, D., Frankel, H., & Gentilello, L. M. (2007). Quantity and quality of sleep in the surgical intensive care unit: Are our patients sleeping? *Journal of Trauma, 63*(6), 1210–1214. Available from https://doi.org/10.1097/TA.0b013e31815b83d700005373-200712000-00003. Retrieved from <http://www.ncbi.nlm.nih.gov/entrez/query.fcgi?cmd = Retrieve&db = PubMed&dopt = Citation&list_uids = 18212640>. [pii].

Gabor, J. Y., Cooper, A. B., & Hanly, P. J. (2001). Sleep disruption in the intensive care unit. *Current Opinion in Critical Care, 7*(1), 21–27. Retrieved from <http://www.ncbi.nlm.nih.gov/entrez/query.fcgi?cmd = Retrieve&db = PubMed&dopt = Citation&list_uids = 11373507>.

Gan, C., Campbell, K. A., Gemeinhardt, M., & McFadden, G. T. (2006). Predictors of family system functioning after brain injury. *Brain Injury, 20*(6), 587–600. Available from https://doi.org/10.1080/02699050600743725.

Giza, C. C., Kutcher, J. S., Ashwal, S., Barth, J., Getchius, T. S., Gioia, G. A., ... Zafonte, R. (2013). Summary of evidence-based guideline update: evaluation and management of concussion in sports: report of the Guideline Development Subcommittee of the American Academy of Neurology. *Neurology, 80*(24), 2250–2257. Available from https://doi.org/10.1212/WNL.0b013e31828d57dd, Epub 2013 Mar 18. Review. PubMed PMID: 23508730; PubMed Central PMCID: PMC3721093.

Giza, C. C., Choe, M. C., & Barlow, K. M. (2018). Determining if rest is best after concussion. *JAMA Neurology, 75*(4), 399–400. Available from https://doi.org/10.1001/jamaneurol.2018.0006.

Gordon, W. A., Sliwinski, M., Echo, J., McLoughlin, M., Sheerer, M. S., & Meili, T. E. (1998). The benefits of exercise in individuals with traumatic brain injury: A retrospective study. *Journal of Head Trauma Rehabilitation, 13*(4), 58–67.

Gould, K. R., Ponsford, J. L., Johnston, L., & Schonberger, M. (2011). The nature, frequency and course of psychiatric disorders in the first year after traumatic brain injury: A prospective study. *Psychological Medicine, 41*(10), 2099–2109. Available from https://doi.org/10.1017/S003329171100033X. Retrieved from <http://www.ncbi.nlm.nih.gov/pubmed/21477420>.

Grauwmeijer, E., Heijenbrok-Kal, M. H., Haitsma, I. K., & Ribbers, G. M. (2017). Employment outcome ten years after moderate to severe traumatic brain injury: A prospective cohort study. *Journal of Neurotrauma, 34*(17), 2575–2581. Available from https://doi.org/10.1089/neu.2016.4846.

Grauwmeijer, E., Heijenbrok-Kal, M. H., Peppel, L. D., Hartjes, C. J., Haitsma, I. K., de Koning, I., & Ribbers, G. M. (2018). Cognition, health-related quality of life, and depression ten years after moderate to severe traumatic brain injury: A prospective cohort study. *Journal of Neurotrauma, 35*(13), 1543–1551. Available from https://doi.org/10.1089/neu.2017.5404.

Grauwmeijer, E., Heijenbrok-Kal, M. H., & Ribbers, G. M. (2014). Health-related quality of life 3 years after moderate to severe traumatic brain injury: A prospective cohort study. *Archives of Physical Medicine and Rehabilitation, 95*(7), 1268–1276. Available from https://doi.org/10.1016/j.apmr.2014.02.002.

Grima, N., Ponsford, J., Rajaratnam, S. M., Mansfield, D., & Pase, M. P. (2016). Sleep disturbances in traumatic brain injury: A meta-analysis. *Journal of Clinical Sleep Medicine*, 12(3), 419−428.

Grima, N. A., Ponsford, J. L., St Hilaire, M. A., Mansfield, D., Rajaratnam, S. M., Grima, N., . . . Pase, M. P. (2016). Circadian melatonin rhythm following traumatic brain injury. *Neurorehabilitation and Neural Repair*, 30(10), 972−977. Available from https://doi.org/ 10.1177/1545968316650279.

Grima, N. A., Rajaratnam, S. M. W., Mansfield, D., Sletten, T. L., Spitz, G., & Ponsford, J. L. (2018). Efficacy of melatonin for sleep disturbance following traumatic brain injury: A randomised controlled trial. *BMC Medicine*, 16(1), 8. Available from https://doi.org/ 10.5664/jcsm.5598.

Gupta, P. K., Sayed, N., Ding, K., Agostini, M. A., Van Ness, P. C., Yablon, S., . . . Diaz-Arrastia, R. (2014). Subtypes of post-traumatic epilepsy: Clinical, electrophysiological, and imaging features. *Journal of Neurotrauma*, 31(16), 1439−1443. Available from https://doi.org/10.1089/neu.2013.3221.

Hall, R. C., Hall, R. C., & Chapman, M. J. (2005). Definition, diagnosis, and forensic implications of postconcussional syndrome. *Psychosomatics*, 46(3), 195−202. Available from https://doi.org/10.1176/appi.psy.46.3.195. Retrieved from <http://www.ncbi.nlm. nih.gov/pubmed/15883140>.

Harvey, A. G. (2005). A cognitive theory and therapy for chronic insomnia. *Journal of Cognitive Psychotherapy*, 19(1), 41−59.

Hauri, P. J. (1991). *Case studies in insomnia*. New York: Plenum Press.

Hesdorffer, D. C., Rauch, S. L., & Tamminga, C. A. (2009). Long-term psychiatric outcomes following traumatic brain injury: A review of the literature. *Journal of Head Trauma Rehabilitation*, 24(6), 452−459. Available from https://doi.org/10.1097/ HTR.0b013e3181c133fd. Retrieved from <http://www.ncbi.nlm.nih.gov/pubmed/ 19940678>.

Hilfiker, R., Meichtry, A., Eicher, M., Nilsson Balfe, L., Knols, R. H., Verra, M. L., & Taeymans, J. (2018). Exercise and other non-pharmaceutical interventions for cancer-related fatigue in patients during or after cancer treatment: A systematic review incorporating an indirect-comparisons meta-analysis. *British Journal of Sports Medicine*, 52 (10), 651−658. Available from https://doi.org/10.1136/bjsports-2016-096422.

Hoffman, J. M., Bell, K. R., Powell, J. M., Behr, J., Dunn, E. C., Dikmen, S., & Bombardier, C. H. (2010). A randomized controlled trial of exercise to improve mood after traumatic brain injury. *PM R*, 2(10), 911−919. Available from https://doi.org/10.1016/j. pmrj.2010.06.008. Retrieved from <http://www.ncbi.nlm.nih.gov/pubmed/20970760>.

Hoofien, D., Gilboa, A., Vakil, E., & Donovick, P. J. (2001). Traumatic brain injury (TBI) 10-20 years later: A comprehensive outcome study of psychiatric symptomatology, cognitive abilities and psychosocial functioning. *Brain Injury*, 15(3), 189−209. Available from https://doi.org/10.1080/026990501300005659. Retrieved from <http://www.ncbi.nlm. nih.gov/pubmed/11260769>.

Horner, M. D., Selassie, A. W., Lineberry, L., Ferguson, P. L., & Labbate, L. A. (2008). Predictors of psychological symptoms 1 year after traumatic brain injury: A population-based, epidemiological study. *Journal of Head Trauma Rehabilitation*, 23(2), 74−83.

Hou, R., Moss-Morris, R., Peveler, R., Mogg, K., Bradley, B. P., & Belli, A. (2012). When a minor head injury results in enduring symptoms: A prospective investigation of risk factors for postconcussional syndrome after mild traumatic brain injury. *Journal of Neurology, Neurosurgery, and Psychiatry*, 83(2), 217−223. Available from https://doi. org/10.1136/jnnp-2011-300767. Retrieved from <http://www.ncbi.nlm.nih.gov/ pubmed/22028384>.

Hutchison, M., Mainwaring, L. M., Comper, P., Richards, D. W., & Bisschop, S. M. (2009). Differential emotional responses of varsity athletes to concussion and musculoskeletal injuries. *Clinical Journal of Sport Medicine*, 19(1), 13−19. Available from https://doi.org/

10.1097/JSM.0b013e318190ba06. Retrieved from <http://www.ncbi.nlm.nih.gov/pubmed/19124978>.

INESSS-ONF. (2016). *Clinical practice guideline for the rehabilitation of adults with moderate to severe traumatic brain injury.* Retrieved from <http://www.braininjuryguidelines.org/>.

Jain, A., Mittal, R. S., Sharma, A., Sharma, A., & Gupta, I. D. (2014). Study of insomnia and associated factors in traumatic brain injury. *Asian Journal of Psychiatry, 8,* 99−103. Available from https://doi.org/10.1016/j.ajp.2013.12.017.

Jha, A., Weintraub, A., Allshouse, A., Morey, C., Cusick, C., Kittelson, J., ... Gerber, D. (2008). A randomized trial of modafinil for the treatment of fatigue and excessive daytime sleepiness in individuals with chronic traumatic brain injury. *Journal of Head Trauma Rehabilitation, 23*(1), 52−63. Available from https://doi.org/10.1097/01.HTR.0000308721.77911.ea.

Johansson, B., & Rönnbäck, L. (2014). Evaluation of the mental fatigue scale and its relation to cognitive and emotional functioning after traumatic brain injury or stroke. *International Journal of Physical Medicine and Rehabilitation, 2*(182), 2.

Johansson, B., & Ronnback, L. (2015). Novel computer tests for identification of mental fatigue after traumatic brain injury. *NeuroRehabilitation.* Available from https://doi.org/10.3233/NRE-151207. Retrieved from <http://www.ncbi.nlm.nih.gov/pubmed/25882202>.

Juengst, S., Skidmore, E., Arenth, P. M., Niyonkuru, C., & Raina, K. D. (2012). The unique contribution of fatigue to disability in community dwelling adults with traumatic brain injury. *Archives of Physical Medicine and Rehabilitation.* Available from https://doi.org/10.1016/j.apmr.2012.07.025. Retrieved from <http://www.ncbi.nlm.nih.gov/pubmed/22885286>.

Kelley, G. A., & Kelley, K. S. (2017). Exercise and sleep: A systematic review of previous meta-analyses. *Journal of Evidence-Based Medicine, 10*(1), 26−36. Available from https://doi.org/10.1111/jebm.12236.

Kempf, J., Werth, E., Kaiser, P. R., Bassetti, C. L., & Baumann, C. R. (2010). Sleep-wake disturbances 3 years after traumatic brain injury. *Journal of Neurology, Neurosurgery, and Psychiatry, 81*(12), 1402−1405. Available from https://doi.org/10.1136/jnnp.2009.201913. Retrieved from <http://www.ncbi.nlm.nih.gov/pubmed/20884672>.

Kersel, D. A., Marsh, N. V., Havill, J. H., & Sleigh, J. W. (2001a). Neuropsychological functioning during the year following severe traumatic brain injury. *Brain Injury, 15*(4), 283−296.

Kersel, D. A., Marsh, N. V., Havill, J. H., & Sleigh, J. W. (2001b). Psychosocial functioning during the year following severe traumatic brain injury. *Brain Injury, 15*(8), 683−696. Available from https://doi.org/10.1080/02699050010013662. Retrieved from <http://www.ncbi.nlm.nih.gov/pubmed/11485609>.

Keyser-Marcus, L. A., Bricout, J. C., Wehman, P., Campbell, L. R., Cifu, D. X., Englander, J., ... Zafonte, R. D. (2002). Acute predictors of return to employment after traumatic brain injury: A longitudinal follow-up. *Archives of Physical Medicine and Rehabilitation, 83*(5), 635−641.

Khoury, S., & Benavides, R. (2017). Pain with traumatic brain injury and psychological disorders. *Progress in Neuro-Psychopharmacology & Biological Psychiatry.* Available from https://doi.org/10.1016/j.pnpbp.2017.06.007. Retrieved from <https://www.ncbi.nlm.nih.gov/pubmed/28627447>.

Khoury, S., Chouchou, F., Amzica, F., Giguere, J. F., Denis, R., Rouleau, G. A., & Lavigne, G. J. (2013). Rapid EEG activity during sleep dominates in mild traumatic brain injury patients with acute pain. *Journal of Neurotrauma, 30*(8), 633−641. Available from https://doi.org/10.1089/neu.2012.2519. Retrieved from <https://www.ncbi.nlm.nih.gov/pubmed/23510169>.

Kolakowsky-Hayner, S. A., Bellon, K., Toda, K., Bushnik, T., Wright, J., Isaac, L., & Englander, J. (2017). A randomised control trial of walking to ameliorate brain injury fatigue: A NIDRR TBI model system centre-based study. *Neuropsychological Rehabilitation*, 27(7), 1002–1018. Available from https://doi.org/10.1080/09602011.2016.1229680.

Koponen, S., Taiminen, T., Hiekkanen, H., & Tenovuo, O. (2011). Axis I and II psychiatric disorders in patients with traumatic brain injury: A 12-month follow-up study. *Brain Injury*, 25(11), 1029–1034. Available from https://doi.org/10.3109/02699052.2011.607783. Retrieved from <http://www.ncbi.nlm.nih.gov/pubmed/21870901>.

Kreber, L. A., Griesbach, G. S., & Ashley, M. J. (2016). Detection of growth hormone deficiency in adults with chronic traumatic brain injury. *Journal of Neurotrauma*, 33(17), 1607–1613. Available from https://doi.org/10.1089/neu.2015.4127.

Kreutzer, J. S., Rapport, L. J., Marwitz, J. H., Harrison-Felix, C., Hart, T., Glenn, M., & Hammond, F. (2009). Caregivers' well-being after traumatic brain injury: A multicenter prospective investigation. *Archives of Physical Medicine and Rehabilitation*, 90(6), 939–946. Available from https://doi.org/10.1016/j.apmr.2009.01.010. Retrieved from <http://www.ncbi.nlm.nih.gov/pubmed/19480869>.

Lamontagne, M. E., Ouellet, M. C., & Simard, J. F. (2009). A descriptive portrait of human assistance required by individuals with brain injury. *Brain Injury*, 23(7), 693–701. Available from https://doi.org/10.1080/02699050902970760. Retrieved from <http://www.ncbi.nlm.nih.gov/pubmed/19557573>.

Larson, E. B., & Zollman, F. S. (2010). The effect of sleep medications on cognitive recovery from traumatic brain injury. *Journal of Head Trauma Rehabilitation*, 25(1), 61–67.

Larun, L., Brurberg, K. G., Odgaard-Jensen, J., & Price, J. R. (2017). Exercise therapy for chronic fatigue syndrome. *Cochrane Database of Systematic Reviews*, 4, Cd003200. Available from https://doi.org/10.1002/14651858.CD003200.pub7.

Lefebvre, H., Cloutier, G., & Levert, M. J. (2008). Perspectives of survivors of traumatic brain injury and their caregivers on long-term social integration. *Brain Injury*, 22(7-8), 535–543. Available from https://doi.org/10.1080/02699050802158243. Retrieved from <http://www.ncbi.nlm.nih.gov/pubmed/18568706>.

Lequerica, A. H., Botticello, A. L., Lengenfelder, J., Chiaravalloti, N., Bushnik, T., Dijkers, M. P., . . . Rosenthal, J. (2017). Factors associated with remission of post-traumatic brain injury fatigue in the years following traumatic brain injury (TBI): A TBI model systems module study. *Neuropsychological Rehabilitation*, 27(7), 1019–1030. Available from https://doi.org/10.1080/09602011.2016.1231120.

Lin, J. M., Brimmer, D. J., Maloney, E. M., Nyarko, E., Belue, R., & Reeves, W. C. (2009). Further validation of the Multidimensional Fatigue Inventory in a US adult population sample. *Population Health Metrics*, 7, 18. Available from https://doi.org/10.1186/1478-7954-7-18. Retrieved from <http://www.ncbi.nlm.nih.gov/pubmed/20003524>.

Losoi, H., Silverberg, N. D., Waljas, M., Turunen, S., Rosti-Otajarvi, E., Helminen, M., . . . Iverson, G. L. (2016). Recovery from mild traumatic brain injury in previously healthy adults. *Journal of Neurotrauma*, 33(8), 766–776. Available from https://doi.org/10.1089/neu.2015.4070.

Lowe, A., Neligan, A., & Greenwood, R. (2019). Sleep disturbance and recovery during rehabilitation after traumatic brain injury: A systematic review. *Disability and Rehabilitation*, 1–14. Available from https://doi.org/10.1080/09638288.2018.1516819.

Lu, W., Krellman, J. W., & Dijkers, M. P. (2016). Can cognitive behavioral therapy for insomnia also treat fatigue, pain, and mood symptoms in individuals with traumatic brain injury?—A multiple case report. *NeuroRehabilitation*, 38(1), 59–69. Available from https://doi.org/10.3233/nre-151296.

Lundin, A., de Boussard, C., Edman, G., & Borg, J. (2006). Symptoms and disability until 3 months after mild TBI. *Brain Injury*, 20(8), 799–806. Available from https://doi.org/10.1080/02699050600744327. Retrieved from <http://www.ncbi.nlm.nih.gov/pubmed/17060147>.

MacMillan, P. J., Hart, R. P., Martelli, M. F., & Zasler, N. D. (2002). Pre-injury status and adaptation following traumatic brain injury. *Brain Injury, 16*(1), 41−49. Available from https://doi.org/10.1080/0269905011008812.

Mahmood, O., Rapport, L. J., Hanks, R. A., & Fichtenberg, N. L. (2004). Neuropsychological performance and sleep disturbance following traumatic brain injury. *Journal of Head Trauma Rehabilitation, 19*(5), 378−390. Retrieved from <http://www.ncbi.nlm.nih.gov/entrez/query.fcgi?cmd = Retrieve&db = PubMed&dopt = Citation&list_uids = 15597029>.

Makley, M. J., Johnson-Greene, L., Tarwater, P. M., Kreuz, A. J., Spiro, J., Rao, V., & Celnik, P. A. (2009). Return of memory and sleep efficiency following moderate to severe closed head injury. *Neurorehabilitation and Neural Repair, 23*(4), 320−326. Retrieved from <http://www.ncbi.nlm.nih.gov/entrez/query.fcgi?cmd = Retrieve &db = PubMed&dopt = Citation&list_uids = 19171947>.

Malec, J. F., Testa, J. A., Rush, B. K., Brown, A. W., & Moessner, A. M. (2007). Self-assessment of impairment, impaired self-awareness, and depression after traumatic brain injury. *Journal of Head Trauma Rehabilitation, 22*(3), 156−166. Available from https://doi.org/10.1097/01.HTR.0000271116.12028.af. Retrieved from <http://www.ncbi.nlm.nih.gov/pubmed/17510591>.

Martelli, M. F., Nicholson, K., & Zasler, N. D. (2013). *Psychological assessment and management of post-traumatic pain. I. Brain injury medicine: Principles and practice* (pp. 974−987). New York: Demos Medical.

Masel, B. E., & DeWitt, D. S. (2010). Traumatic brain injury: A disease process, not an event. *Journal of Neurotrauma, 27*(8), 1529−1540. Available from https://doi.org/10.1089/neu.2010.1358. Retrieved from <http://www.ncbi.nlm.nih.gov/pubmed/20504161>.

Mathias, J. L., & Alvaro, P. K. (2012). Prevalence of sleep disturbances, disorders, and problems following traumatic brain injury: A meta-analysis. *Sleep Medicine, 13*(7), 898−905. Available from https://doi.org/10.1016/j.sleep.2012.04.006. Retrieved from <http://www.ncbi.nlm.nih.gov/pubmed/22705246>.

McBrinn, J., Colin Wilson, F., Caldwell, S., Carton, S., Delargy, M., McCann, J., ... McGuire, B. (2008). Emotional distress and awareness following acquired brain injury: An exploratory analysis. *Brain Injury, 22*(10), 765−772. Available from https://doi.org/10.1080/02699050802372208. Retrieved from <http://www.ncbi.nlm.nih.gov/pubmed/18787986>.

McCrimmon, S., & Oddy, M. (2006). Return to work following moderate-to-severe traumatic brain injury. *Brain Injury, 20*(10), 1037−1046. Available from https://doi.org/10.1080/02699050600909656. Retrieved from <http://www.ncbi.nlm.nih.gov/pubmed/17060136>.

Meares, S., Shores, E. A., Taylor, A. J., Batchelor, J., Bryant, R. A., Baguley, I. J., ... Marosszeky, J. E. (2011). The prospective course of postconcussion syndrome: The role of mild traumatic brain injury. *Neuropsychology, 25*(4), 454−465. Available from https://doi.org/10.1037/a0022580. Retrieved from <http://www.ncbi.nlm.nih.gov/pubmed/21574719>.

Menon, D. K., Schwab, K., Wright, D. W., & Maas, A. I. (2010). Position statement: Definition of traumatic brain injury. *Archives of Physical Medicine and Rehabilitation, 91* (11), 1637−1640. Available from https://doi.org/10.1016/j.apmr.2010.05.017.

Moldofsky, H. (1989). Sleep influences on regional and diffuse pain syndromes associated with osteoarthritis. *Seminars in Arthritis and Rheumatism, 18*(4 Suppl. 2), 18−21. Retrieved from <http://www.ncbi.nlm.nih.gov/entrez/query.fcgi?cmd = Retrieve &db = PubMed&dopt = Citation&list_uids = 2658072>.

Mollayeva, T., Kendzerska, T., Mollayeva, S., Shapiro, C. M., Colantonio, A., & Cassidy, J. D. (2014). A systematic review of fatigue in patients with traumatic brain injury: The course, predictors and consequences. *Neuroscience and Biobehavioral Reviews, 47*, 684−716. Available from https://doi.org/10.1016/j.neubiorev.2014.10.024. Retrieved from <http://www.ncbi.nlm.nih.gov/pubmed/25451201>.

Mollayeva, T., Mollayeva, S., Shapiro, C. M., Cassidy, J. D., & Colantonio, A. (2016). Insomnia in workers with delayed recovery from mild traumatic brain injury. *Sleep Medicine, 19*, 153–161. Available from https://doi.org/10.1016/j.sleep.2015.05.014.

Mollayeva, T., Shapiro, C. M., Mollayeva, S., Cassidy, J. D., & Colantonio, A. (2015). Modeling community integration in workers with delayed recovery from mild traumatic brain injury. *BMC Neurology, 15*, 194. Available from https://doi.org/10.1186/s12883-015-0432-z.

Morin, C., LeBlanc, M., Belanger, L., Ivers, H., Merette, C., & Savard, J. (2011). Prevalence of insomnia and its treatment in Canada. *Canadian Journal of Psychiatry, 56*(9), 540–548. Retrieved from <http://www.ncbi.nlm.nih.gov/entrez/query.fcgi?cmd = Retrieve&db = PubMed&dopt = Citation&list_uids = 21959029>.

Morin, C. M. (1993). *Insomnia: Psychological assessment and management*. New York: Guilford.

Morin, C. M., LeBlanc, M., Daley, M., Gregoire, J. P., & Merette, C. (2006). Epidemiology of insomnia: Prevalence, self-help treatments, consultations, and determinants of help-seeking behaviors. *Sleep Medicine, 7*(2), 123–130. Available from https://doi.org/10.1016/j.sleep.2005.08.008. Retrieved from <https://www.ncbi.nlm.nih.gov/pubmed/16459140>.

Morin, C. M., Vallieres, A., & Ivers, H. (2007). Dysfunctional beliefs and attitudes about sleep (DBAS): Validation of a brief version (DBAS-16). *Sleep, 30*(11), 1547–1554.

Morris, T. (2010). Traumatic brain injury. 17-32. https://doi.org/10.1007/978-1-4419-1364-7_2

Morton, M., & Wehman, P. (1995). Psychosocial and emotional sequelae of individuals with traumatic brain injury: A literature review and recommendations. *Brain Injury, 9* (1), 81–92.

Moye, L. S., & Pradhan, A. A. (2017). From blast to bench: A translational mini-review of posttraumatic headache. *Journal of Neuroscience Research, 95*(6), 1347–1354. Available from https://doi.org/10.1002/jnr.24001. Retrieved from <https://www.ncbi.nlm.nih.gov/pubmed/28151589>.

Nampiaparampil, D. E. (2008). Prevalence of chronic pain after traumatic brain injury: A systematic review. *The Journal of the American Medical Association, 300*(6), 711–719. Available from https://doi.org/10.1001/jama.300.6.711. Retrieved from <http://www.ncbi.nlm.nih.gov/pubmed/18698069>.

National Institutes of Health. (2005). National Institutes of Health State of the Science conference statement on manifestations and management of chronic insomnia in adults, June 13-15, 2005. *Sleep, 28*(9), 1049–1057. Retrieved from <http://www.ncbi.nlm.nih.gov/entrez/query.fcgi?cmd = Retrieve&db = PubMed&dopt = Citation&list_uids = 16268373>.

Nguyen, S., McKay, A., Wong, D., Rajaratnam, S. M., Spitz, G., Williams, G., ... Ponsford, J. L. (2017). Cognitive behavior therapy to treat sleep disturbance and fatigue after traumatic brain injury: A pilot randomized controlled trial. *Archives of Physical Medicine and Rehabilitation, 98* (8). Available from https://doi.org/10.1016/j.apmr.2017.02.031, 1508.e2-1517.e2.

Nguyen, S., McKenzie, D., McKay, A., Wong, D., Rajaratnam, S. M. W., Spitz, G., ... Ponsford, J. L. (2018). Exploring predictors of treatment outcome in cognitive behavior therapy for sleep disturbance following acquired brain injury. *Disability and Rehabilitation, 40*(16), 1906–1913. Available from https://doi.org/10.1080/09638288.2017.131546110.1016/j.apmr.2017.02.031.

Nguyen, S., Wong, D., McKay, A., Rajaratnam, S. M. W., Spitz, G., Williams, G., ... Ponsford, J. L. (2019). Cognitive behavioural therapy for post-stroke fatigue and sleep disturbance: A pilot randomised controlled trial with blind assessment. *Neuropsychological Rehabilitation, 29*(5), 723–738. Available from https://doi.org/10.1080/09602011.2017.1326945.

NICE. (2007). *Chronic fatigue syndrome/myalgic encephalomyelitis (or encephalopathy): Diagnosis and management (Clinical Guideline CG53)*. Retrieved from <https://www.nice.org.uk/guidance/cg53>.

Norrie, J., Heitger, M., Leathem, J., Anderson, T., Jones, R., & Flett, R. (2010). Mild traumatic brain injury and fatigue: A prospective longitudinal study. *Brain Injury, 24* (13–14), 1528–1538. Available from https://doi.org/10.3109/02699052.2010.531687. Retrieved from <http://www.ncbi.nlm.nih.gov/pubmed/21058899>.

Novack, T. A., Labbe, D., Grote, M., Carlson, N., Sherer, M., Arango-Lasprilla, J. C., . . . Seel, R. T. (2010). Return to driving within 5 years of moderate-severe traumatic brain injury. *Brain Injury, 24*(3), 464–471. Available from https://doi.org/10.3109/02699051003601713. Retrieved from <http://www.ncbi.nlm.nih.gov/pubmed/20184403>.

Ohayon, M. M. (2002). Epidemiology of insomnia: What we know and what we still need to learn. *Sleep Medicine Reviews, 6*(2), 97–111.

Olver, J. H., Ponsford, J. L., & Curran, C. A. (1996). Outcome following traumatic brain injury: A comparison between 2 and 5 years after injury. *Brain Injury, 10*(11), 841–848. Available from https://doi.org/10.1080/026990596123945. Retrieved from <http://www.ncbi.nlm.nih.gov/entrez/query.fcgi?cmd = Retrieve&db = PubMed&dopt = Citation&list_uids = 8905161>.

ONF. (2018). *Guideline for concussion/mild traumatic brain injury & persistent symptoms, 3rd edition, for adults over 18 years of age.* Retrieved from <https://braininjuryguidelines. org/concussion/>.

O'Shanick, G.J., & O'Shanick, A. (2005). *Personality disorders.* In J. Silver, T. McAllister, & S. Yudofsky (Eds.), Textbook of traumatic brain injury. (pp. 245-258). Washington, DC: American Psychiatric Publishing.

O'Shanick, G.J., O'Shanick, A., & Znotens, J. (2011). *Personality change.* In J. Silver, T. McAllister & S. Yudofsky (Eds.). *Textbook of traumatic brain injury, 2nd Edition.* (pp. 211–223). Washington, DC: American Psychiatric Publishing.

Osier, N. D., Pham, L., Pugh, B. J., Puccio, A., Ren, D., Conley, Y. P., . . . Dixon, C. E. (2017). Brain injury results in lower levels of melatonin receptors subtypes MT1 and MT2. *Neuroscience Letters, 650,* 18–24.

Ouellet, M., Beaulieu-Bonneau, S., & Morin, C. (2006). Insomnia in patients with traumatic brain injury: Frequency, characteristics, and risk factors. *Journal of Head Trauma Rehabilitation, 21*(3), 199–212.

Ouellet, M.-C., Beaulieu-Bonneau, S., & Morin, C. M. (2012). Sleep-wake disturbances and fatigue in brain-injured individuals. In C. A. Espie, & C. M. Morin (Eds.), *Oxford handbook of sleep and sleep disorders* (pp. 820–845). Oxford: Oxford University Press.

Ouellet, M.-C., Beaulieu-Bonneau, S., & Morin, C. M. (2015). Sleep-wake disturbances after traumatic brain injury. *The Lancet Neurology, 14*(7), 746–757. Available from https:// doi.org/10.1016/s1474-4422(15)00068-x.

Ouellet, M.-C., & Morin, C. M. (2004). Cognitive behavioral therapy for insomnia associated with traumatic brain injury: A single-case study. *Archives of Physical Medicine and Rehabilitation, 85*(8), 1298–1302. Available from https://doi.org/10.1016/j. apmr.2003.11.036. Retrieved from <http://www.ncbi.nlm.nih.gov/pubmed/15295756>.

Ouellet, M.-C., & Morin, C. M. (2006). Fatigue following traumatic brain injury: Frequency, characteristics, and associated factors. *Rehabilitation Psychology, 51*(2), 140–149.

Ouellet, M.-C., & Morin, C. M. (2007). Efficacy of cognitive-behavioral therapy for insomnia associated with traumatic brain injury: A single-case experimental design. *Archives of Physical Medicine and Rehabilitation, 88*(12), 1581–1592. Available from https://doi.org/ 10.1016/j.apmr.2007.09.006. Retrieved from <http://www.ncbi.nlm.nih.gov/entrez/ query.fcgi?cmd = Retrieve&db = PubMed&dopt = Citation&list_uids = 18047872>.

Ouellet, M.-C., Morin, C. M., & Lavoie, A. (2009). Volunteer work and psychological health following traumatic brain injury. *Journal of Head Trauma Rehabilitation, 24*(4), 262–271. Available from https://doi.org/10.1097/HTR.0b013e3181a68b73. Retrieved from <http://www.ncbi.nlm.nih.gov/pubmed/19625865>.

Ouellet, M.-C., Savard, J., & Morin, C. M. (2004). Insomnia following traumatic brain injury: A review. *Neurorehabilitation and Neural Repair, 18*(4), 187–198. Available from https://doi.org/10.1177/1545968304271405. Retrieved from <http://www.ncbi.nlm.nih.gov/entrez/query.fcgi?cmd = Retrieve&db = PubMed&dopt = Citation&list_uids = 15669131>.

Pagulayan, K. F., Hoffman, J. M., Temkin, N. R., Machamer, J. E., & Dikmen, S. S. (2008). Functional limitations and depression after traumatic brain injury: Examination of the temporal relationship. *Archives of Physical Medicine and Rehabilitation, 89*(10), 1887−1892. Available from https://doi.org/10.1016/j.apmr.2008.03.019. Retrieved from <http://www.ncbi.nlm.nih.gov/pubmed/18929017>.

Paparrigopoulos, T., Melissaki, A., Tsekou, H., Efthymiou, A., Kribeni, G., Baziotis, N., & Geronikola, X. (2006). Melatonin secretion after head injury: A pilot study. *Brain Injury, 20*(8), 873−878.

Parcell, D. L., Ponsford, J. L., Rajaratnam, S. M., & Redman, J. R. (2006). Self-reported changes to nighttime sleep after traumatic brain injury. *Archives of Physical Medicine and Rehabilitation, 87*(2), 278−285. Retrieved from <http://www.ncbi.nlm.nih.gov/entrez/query.fcgi?cmd = Retrieve&db = PubMed&dopt = Citation&list_uids = 16442985>.

Parcell, D. L., Ponsford, J. L., Redman, J. R., & Rajaratnam, S. M. (2008). Poor sleep quality and changes in objectively recorded sleep after traumatic brain injury: A preliminary study. *Archives of Physical Medicine and Rehabilitation, 89*(5), 843−850. Available from https://doi.org/10.1016/j.apmr.2007.09.057. Retrieved from <http://www.ncbi.nlm.nih.gov/entrez/query.fcgi?cmd = Retrieve&db = PubMed&dopt = Citation&list_uids = 18452730>.

Perlis, M., & Buysse, D. J. (2011). Pathophysiology and models of insomnia. In M. H. Kryger, T. Roth, & W. C. Dement (Eds.), *Principles and practice of sleep medicine* (5th ed.). Philadelphia: PA: Saunders.

Perlis, M. L., Artiola, L., & Giles, D. E. (1997). Sleep complaints in chronic postconcussion syndrome. *Perceptual and Motor Skills, 84*(2), 595−599. Retrieved from <http://www.ncbi.nlm.nih.gov/entrez/query.fcgi?cmd = Retrieve&db = PubMed&dopt = Citation&list_uids = 9106853>.

Pigeon, W. R., Sateia, M. J., & Ferguson, R. J. (2003). Distinguishing between excessive daytime sleepiness and fatigue: Toward improved detection and treatment. *Journal of Psychosomatic Research, 54*, 61−69. Available from https://doi.org/10.1016/S0022-3999 (02)00542-1.

Polinder, S., Haagsma, J. A., van Klaveren, D., Steyerberg, E. W., & van Beeck, E. F. (2015). Health-related quality of life after TBI: A systematic review of study design, instruments, measurement properties, and outcome. *Population Health Metrics, 13*, 4. Available from https://doi.org/10.1186/s12963-015-0037-1.

Ponsford, J., Nguyen, S., Downing, M., Bosch, M., McKenzie, J. E., Turner, S., . . . Green, S. (2019). Factors associated with persistent post-concussion symptoms following mild traumatic brain injury in adults. *Journal of Rehabilitation Medicine, 51*(1), 32−39. Available from https://doi.org/10.2340/16501977-2492.

Ponsford, J., & Ziino, C. (2003). Fatigue and attention following traumatic brain injury [Abstract]. *Zeitschrift für Neuropsychologie, 14*, 155−163.

Ponsford, J., Ziino, C., Parcell, D. L., Shekleton, J. A., Roper, M., Redman, J. R., . . . Rajaratnam, S. M. (2012). Fatigue and sleep disturbance following traumatic brain injury—their nature, causes, and potential treatments. *Journal of Head Trauma Rehabilitation, 27*(3), 224−233. Available from https://doi.org/10.1097/HTR.0b013e31824ee1a8. Retrieved from <http://www.ncbi.nlm.nih.gov/pubmed/22573041>.

Ponsford, J. L., Downing, M. G., Olver, J., Ponsford, M., Acher, R., Carty, M., & Spitz, G. (2014). Longitudinal follow-up of patients with traumatic brain injury: Outcome at two, five, and ten years post-injury. *Journal of Neurotrauma, 31*(1), 64−77. Available from https://doi.org/10.1089/neu.2013.2997.

Price, J. R., Mitchell, E., Tidy, E., & Hunot, V. (2008). Cognitive behaviour therapy for chronic fatigue syndrome in adults. *Cochrane Database of Systematic Reviews* (3),

CD001027. Available from https://doi.org/10.1002/14651858.CD001027.pub2. Retrieved from <http://www.ncbi.nlm.nih.gov/entrez/query.fcgi?cmd = Retrieve &db = PubMed&dopt = Citation&list_uids = 18646067>.

Prigatano, G. P. (2005). Disturbances of self-awareness and rehabilitation of patients with traumatic brain injury: A 20-year perspective. *Journal of Head Trauma Rehabilitation, 20* (1), 19−29. Available from https://doi.org/00001199-200501000-00004. Retrieved from [pii] <http://www.ncbi.nlm.nih.gov/pubmed/15668568>.

Ragnarsson, K., Clarke, W., Daling, J., Garber, S., Gustafson, C., Holland, A., . . . Roth, E. (1999). Rehabilitation of persons with traumatic brain injury. *Journal of the American Medical Association, 282*(10), 974−983.

Rao, V., Spiro, J., Vaishnavi, S., Rastogi, P., Mielke, M., Noll, K., . . . Makley, M. (2008). Prevalence and types of sleep disturbances acutely after traumatic brain injury. *Brain Injury, 22*(5), 381−386. Available from https://doi.org/10.1080/02699050801935260. Retrieved from <http://www.ncbi.nlm.nih.gov/entrez/query.fcgi?cmd = Retrieve &db = PubMed&dopt = Citation&list_uids = 18415718>. 792140897 [pii].

Richardson, C., McKay, A., & Ponsford, J. L. (2015). Factors influencing self-awareness following traumatic brain injury. *Journal of Head Trauma Rehabilitation, 30*(2), E43−54. Available from https://doi.org/10.1097/HTR.0000000000000048. Retrieved from <http://www.ncbi.nlm.nih.gov/pubmed/24721809>.

Riese, H., Hoedemaeker, M., Brouwer, W. H., & Mulder, L. J. M. (1999). Mental fatigue after very severe closed head injury: Sustained performance, mental effort, and distress at two levels of workload in a driving simulator. *Neuropsychological Rehabilitation, 9*(2), 189−205. Available from https://doi.org/10.1080/713755600.

Roth, T., Jaeger, S., Jin, R., Kalsekar, A., Stang, P. E., & Kessler, R. C. (2006). Sleep problems, comorbid mental disorders, and role functioning in the national comorbidity survey replication. *Biological Psychiatry, 60*(12), 1364−1371. Available from https://doi.org/10.1016/ j.biopsych.2006.05.039. Retrieved from <http://www.ncbi.nlm.nih.gov/entrez/query. fcgi?cmd = Retrieve&db = PubMed&dopt = Citation&list_uids = 16952333>.

Ruff, R. L., Ruff, S. S., & Wang, X. F. (2009). Improving sleep: Initial headache treatment in OIF/OEF veterans with blast-induced mild traumatic brain injury. *Journal of Rehabilitation Research & Development, 46*(9), 1071−1084. Retrieved from <http://www. ncbi.nlm.nih.gov/pubmed/20437313>.

Schiehser, D. M., Twamley, E. W., Liu, L., Matevosyan, A., Filoteo, J. V., Jak, A. J., . . . Delano-Wood, L. (2015). The relationship between postconcussive symptoms and quality of life in veterans with mild to moderate traumatic brain injury. *Journal of Head Trauma Rehabilitation, 30*(4), E21−28. Available from https://doi.org/10.1097/ htr.0000000000000065.

Schonberger, M., Herrberg, M., & Ponsford, J. (2014). Fatigue as a cause, not a consequence of depression and daytime sleepiness: A cross-lagged analysis. *Journal of Head Trauma Rehabilitation, 29*(5), 427−431. Available from https://doi.org/10.1097/ HTR.0b013e31829ddd08.

Shekleton, J. A., Parcell, D. L., Redman, J. R., Phipps-Nelson, J., Ponsford, J. L., & Rajaratnam, S. M. (2010). Sleep disturbance and melatonin levels following traumatic brain injury. *Neurology, 74*(21), 1732−1738. Available from https://doi.org/10.1212/ WNL.0b013e3181e0438b. Retrieved from <http://www.ncbi.nlm.nih.gov/pubmed/ 20498441>.

Shen, J., Barbera, J., & Shapiro, C. M. (2006). Distinguishing sleepiness and fatigue: Focus on definition and measurement. *Sleep Medicine Reviews, 10*(1), 63−76. Retrieved from <http://www.ncbi.nlm.nih.gov/entrez/query.fcgi?cmd = Retrieve&db = PubMed &dopt = Citation&list_uids = 16376590>.

Sherer, M., Yablon, S. A., & Nakase-Richardson, R. (2009). Patterns of recovery of posttraumatic confusional state in neurorehabilitation admissions after traumatic brain injury.

Archives of Physical Medicine and Rehabilitation, 90(10), 1749–1754. Available from https://doi.org/10.1016/j.apmr.2009.05.011.

Sidaros, A., Skimminge, A., Liptrot, M. G., Sidaros, K., Engberg, A. W., Herning, M., ... Rostrup, E. (2009). Long-term global and regional brain volume changes following severe traumatic brain injury: A longitudinal study with clinical correlates. *Neuroimage, 44*(1), 1–8. Available from https://doi.org/10.1016/j.neuroimage.2008.08.030. Retrieved from <http://www.ncbi.nlm.nih.gov/entrez/query.fcgi?cmd = Retrieve &db = PubMed&dopt = Citation&list_uids = 18804539>.

Sigurdardottir, S., Andelic, N., Roe, C., & Schanke, A. K. (2013). Depressive symptoms and psychological distress during the first five years after traumatic brain injury: Relationship with psychosocial stressors, fatigue and pain. *Journal of Rehabilitation Medicine, 45*(8), 808–814. Available from https://doi.org/10.2340/16501977-1156. Retrieved from <http://www.ncbi.nlm.nih.gov/pubmed/24002318>.

Silver, J. M., McAllister, T. W., & Yudofsky, S. C. (Eds.), (2005). *Textbook of traumatic brain injury*. Washington, DC: American Psychiatric Publishing.

Silverberg, N. D., Gardner, A. J., Brubacher, J. R., Panenka, W. J., Li, J. J., & Iverson, G. L. (2015). Systematic review of multivariable prognostic models for mild traumatic brain injury. *Journal of Neurotrauma, 32*(8), 517–526. Available from https://doi.org/10.1089/neu.2014.3600.

Sinclair, K. L., Ponsford, J. L., Taffe, J., Lockley, S. W., & Rajaratnam, S. M. (2014). Randomized controlled trial of light therapy for fatigue following traumatic brain injury. *Neurorehabilitation and Neural Repair, 28*(4), 303–313. Available from https://doi.org/10.1177/1545968313508472, Epub 1545968313502013 Nov 1545968313508478.

Sinnakaruppan, I., & Williams, D. M. (2001). Family carers and the adult head-injured: A critical review of carers' needs. *Brain Injury, 15*(8), 653–672. Available from https://doi.org/10.1080/02699050010025759. Retrieved from <http://www.ncbi.nlm.nih.gov/pubmed/11485607>.

Sirois, M. J., Emond, M., Ouellet, M. C., Perry, J., Daoust, R., Morin, J., ... Allain-Boule, N. (2013). Cumulative incidence of functional decline after minor injuries in previously independent older Canadian individuals in the emergency department. *Journal of the American Geriatrics Society, 61*(10), 1661–1668. Available from https://doi.org/10.1111/jgs.12482.

Smets, E. M., Garssen, B., Bonke, B., & De Haes, J. C. (1995). The Multidimensional Fatigue Inventory (MFI) psychometric qualities of an instrument to assess fatigue. *Journal of Psychosomatic Research, 39*(3), 315–325.

Sommerauer, M., Valko, P. O., Werth, E., & Baumann, C. R. (2013). Excessive sleep need following traumatic brain injury: A case-control study of 36 patients. *Journal of Sleep Research, 22*(6), 634–639. Available from https://doi.org/10.1111/jsr.12068.

Spielman, A. J., Saskin, P., & Thorpy, M. J. (1987). Treatment of chronic insomnia by restriction of time in bed. *Sleep, 10*(1), 45–56. Retrieved from <http://www.ncbi.nlm.nih.gov/entrez/query.fcgi?cmd = Retrieve&db = PubMed&dopt = Citation&list_uids = 3563247>.

Stein, M. B., Ursano, R. J., Campbell-Sills, L., Colpe, L. J., Fullerton, C. S., Heeringa, S. G., ... Kessler, R. C. (2016). Prognostic indicators of persistent post-concussive symptoms after deployment-related mild traumatic brain injury: A prospective longitudinal study in U.S. Army Soldiers. *Journal of Neurotrauma*. Available from https://doi.org/10.1089/neu.2015.4320.

Stulemeijer, M., van der Werf, S., Borm, G. F., & Vos, P. E. (2008). Early prediction of favourable recovery 6 months after mild traumatic brain injury. *Journal of Neurology, Neurosurgery, and Psychiatry, 79*(8), 936–942. Available from https://doi.org/10.1136/jnnp.2007.131250.

Sundstrom, A., Nilsson, L. G., Cruts, M., Adolfsson, R., Van Broeckhoven, C., & Nyberg, L. (2007). Fatigue before and after mild traumatic brain injury: Pre-post-injury comparisons in relation to apolipoprotein E. *Brain Injury, 21*(10), 1049−1054. Available from https://doi.org/10.1080/02699050701630367. Retrieved from <http://www.ncbi. nlm.nih.gov/entrez/query.fcgi?cmd = Retrieve&db = PubMed&dopt = Citation&list_ uids = 17891567>.

Tagliaferri, F., Compagnone, C., Korsic, M., Servadei, F., & Kraus, J. (2006). A systematic review of brain injury epidemiology in Europe. *Acta Neurochir (Wien), 148*(3), 255−268. Available from https://doi.org/10.1007/s00701-005-0651-y, Retrieved from. Available from http://www.ncbi.nlm.nih.gov/pubmed/16311842.

Taylor, C. A., Bell, J. M., Breiding, M. J., & Xu, L. (2017). Traumatic brain injury-related emergency department visits, hospitalizations, and deaths—United States, 2007 and 2013. *MMWR Surveillance Summaries, 66*(9), 1−16. Available from https://doi.org/ 10.15585/mmwr.ss6609a1.

Testa, J. A., Malec, J. F., Moessner, A. M., & Brown, A. W. (2005). Outcome after traumatic brain injury: Effects of aging on recovery. *Archives of Physical Medicine and Rehabilitation, 86*(9), 1815−1823. Available from https://doi.org/10.1016/j.apmr.2005.03.010. Retrieved from <http://www.ncbi.nlm.nih.gov/pubmed/16181948>.

Testa, J. A., Malec, J. F., Moessner, A. M., & Brown, A. W. (2006). Predicting family functioning after TBI: Impact of neurobehavioral factors. *Journal of Head Trauma Rehabilitation, 21*(3), 236−247. Retrieved from <http://www.ncbi.nlm.nih.gov/ pubmed/16717501>.

Theadom, A., Barker-Collo, S., Jones, K., Dudley, M., Vincent, N., Feigin, V., ... McPherson, K. (2018). A pilot randomized controlled trial of on-line interventions to improve sleep quality in adults after mild or moderate traumatic brain injury. *Clinical Rehabilitation, 32*(5), 619−629. Available from https://doi.org/10.1177/ 0269215517736671.

Theadom, A., Cropley, M., Parmar, P., Barker-Collo, S., Starkey, N., Jones, K., ... Group, B.R. (2015). Sleep difficulties one year following mild traumatic brain injury in a population-based study. *Sleep Medicine, 16*(8), 926−932. Available from https://doi.org/10.1016/j. sleep.2015.04.013. Retrieved from <https://www.ncbi.nlm.nih.gov/pubmed/26138280>.

Theadom, A., Rowland, V., Levack, W., Starkey, N., Wilkinson-Meyers, L., & McPherson, K. (2016). Exploring the experience of sleep and fatigue in male and female adults over the 2 years following traumatic brain injury: A qualitative descriptive study. *BMJ Open, 6*(4), e010453. Available from https://doi.org/10.1136/bmjopen-2015-010453.

Toglia, J. P., & Golisz, K. (2012). *Therapy for activities of daily living: Theoretical and practical perspectives. Brain injury medicine.* New York: Demos Medical Publishing.

Trevena, L., & Cameron, I. (2011). Traumatic brain injury: Long term care of patients in general practice. *Australian Family Physician, 40*(12), 956.

VA/DoD. (2016). *Clinical practice guideline for the management of concussion−mild traumatic brain injury.* Washington, DC.

Valko, P. O., Gavrilov, Y. V., Yamamoto, M., Finn, K., Reddy, H., Haybaeck, J., ... Baumann, C. R. (2015). Damage to histaminergic tuberomammillary neurons and other hypothalamic neurons with traumatic brain injury. *Annals of Neurology, 77*(1), 177−182. Available from https://doi.org/10.1002/ana.24298.

van der Naalt, J., van Zomeren, A. H., Sluiter, W. J., & Minderhoud, J. M. (1999). One year outcome in mild to moderate head injury: The predictive value of acute injury characteristics related to complaints and return to work. *Journal of Neurology, Neurosurgery, and Psychiatry, 66*(2), 207−213.

van Zomeren, A. H., Brouwer, W. H., & Deelman, B. G. (1984). Attentional deficits: The riddles of selectivity, speed and alertness. In N. Brooks (Ed.), *Closed head injury: Social and family consequences* (pp. 74−107). Oxford, England: Oxford University Press.

Viola-Saltzman, M., & Watson, N. F. (2012). Traumatic brain injury and sleep disorders. *Neurologic Clinics, 30*(4), 1299−1312. Available from https://doi.org/10.1016/j. ncl.2012.08.008. Retrieved from <https://www.ncbi.nlm.nih.gov/pubmed/23099139>.

Vos-Vromans, D. C., Smeets, R. J., Rijnders, L. J., Gorrissen, R. R., Pont, M., Koke, A. J., ... Knottnerus, A. J. (2012). Cognitive behavioural therapy versus multidisciplinary rehabilitation treatment for patients with chronic fatigue syndrome: Study protocol for a randomised controlled trial (FatiGo). *Trials*, *13*, 71. Available from https://doi.org/10.1186/1745-6215-13-71. Retrieved from <http://www.ncbi.nlm.nih.gov/pubmed/22647321>.

Vuletic, S., Bell, K. R., Jain, S., Bush, N., Temkin, N., Fann, J. R., ... Gahm, G. A. (2016). CONTACT Investigators. Telephone Problem-Solving Treatment Improves Sleep Quality in Service Members With Combat-Related Mild Traumatic Brain Injury: Results From a Randomized Clinical Trial. *J Head Trauma Rehabil*, *31*(2), 147–157. Available from https://doi.org/10.1097/HTR.0000000000000221, PubMed PMID: 26959668.

Vynorius, K. C., Paquin, A. M., & Seichepine, D. R. (2016). Lifetime multiple mild traumatic brain injuries are associated with cognitive and mood symptoms in young healthy college students. *Frontiers in Neurology*, *7*, 188. Available from https://doi.org/10.3389/fneur.2016.00188.

Waldron-Perrine, B., McGuire, A. P., Spencer, R. J., Drag, L. L., Pangilinan, P. H., & Bieliauskas, L. A. (2012). The influence of sleep and mood on cognitive functioning among veterans being evaluated for mild traumatic brain injury. *Military Medicine*, *177*(11), 1293–1301.

Waljas, M., Lange, R. T., Hakulinen, U., Huhtala, H., Dastidar, P., Hartikainen, K., ... Iverson, G. L. (2014). Biopsychosocial outcome after uncomplicated mild traumatic brain injury. *Journal of Neurotrauma*, *31*(1), 108–124. Available from https://doi.org/10.1089/neu.2013.2941. Retrieved from <http://www.ncbi.nlm.nih.gov/pubmed/23978227>, <http://online.liebertpub.com/doi/pdfplus/10.1089/neu.2013.2941>.

Ward, N., & Winters, S. (2003). Results of a fatigue management programme in multiple sclerosis. *British Journal of Nursing*, *12*(18), 1075–1080. Retrieved from <http://www.ncbi.nlm.nih.gov/entrez/query.fcgi?cmd = Retrieve&db = PubMed&dopt = Citation&list_uids = 14581840>.

Webb, W. B., & Agnew, H. W., Jr. (1975). Sleep efficiency for sleep-wake cycles of varied length. *Psychophysiology*, *12*(6), 637–641.

Wessely, S., David, A., Butler, S., & Chalder, T. (1989). Management of chronic (post-viral) fatigue syndrome. *The Journal of the Royal College of General Practitioners*, *39*(318), 26–29.

Whelan-Goodinson, R., Ponsford, J., Johnston, L., & Grant, F. (2009). Psychiatric disorders following traumatic brain injury: Their nature and frequency. *Journal of Head Trauma Rehabilitation*, *24*(5), 324–332. Available from https://doi.org/10.1097/HTR.0b013e3181a712aa. Retrieved from <http://www.ncbi.nlm.nih.gov/pubmed/19858966>.

Whelan-Goodinson, R., Ponsford, J. L., Schonberger, M., & Johnston, L. (2010). Predictors of psychiatric disorders following traumatic brain injury. *Journal of Head Trauma Rehabilitation*, *25*(5), 320–329. Available from https://doi.org/10.1097/HTR.0b013e3181c8f8e7. Retrieved from <http://www.ncbi.nlm.nih.gov/pubmed/20042983>.

Wilson, S. J., Nutt, D. J., Alford, C., Argyropoulos, S. V., Baldwin, D. S., Bateson, A. N., ... Wade, A. G. (2010). British Association for Psychopharmacology consensus statement on evidence-based treatment of insomnia, parasomnias and circadian rhythm disorders. *Journal of Psychopharmacology*, *24*(11), 1577–1601. Available from https://doi.org/10.1177/0269881110379307. Retrieved from <http://www.ncbi.nlm.nih.gov/pubmed/20813762>.

Wiseman-Hakes, C., Murray, B., Moineddin, R., Rochon, E., Cullen, N., Gargaro, J., & Colantonio, A. (2013). Evaluating the impact of treatment for sleep/wake disorders on recovery of cognition and communication in adults with chronic TBI. *Brain Injury*, *27*(12), 1364–1376. Available from https://doi.org/10.3109/02699052.2013.823663.

Wiseman-Hakes, C., Victor, J. C., Brandys, C., & Murray, B. J. (2011). Impact of post-traumatic hypersomnia on functional recovery of cognition and communication. *Brain Injury*, *25*(12), 1256–1265. Available from https://doi.org/10.3109/02699052.2011.608215. Retrieved from <http://www.ncbi.nlm.nih.gov/pubmed/21961569>.

Worthington, A. D., & Melia, Y. (2006). Rehabilitation is compromised by arousal and sleep disorders: Results of a survey of rehabilitation centres. *Brain Injury*, *20*(3), 327–332. Available from https://doi.org/10.1080/02699050500488249. Retrieved from <http://www.ncbi.nlm.nih.gov/entrez/query.fcgi?cmd = Retrieve&db = PubMed&dopt = Citation&list_uids = 16537274>.

Wylie, G. R., Dobryakova, E., DeLuca, J., Chiaravalloti, N., Essad, K., & Genova, H. (2017). Cognitive fatigue in individuals with traumatic brain injury is associated with caudate activation. *Scientific Reports*, *7*(1), 8973. Available from https://doi.org/10.1038/s41598-017-08846-6.

Wylie, G. R., & Flashman, L. A. (2017). Understanding the interplay between mild traumatic brain injury and cognitive fatigue: Models and treatments. *Concussion*, *2*(4), Cnc50. Available from https://doi.org/10.2217/cnc-2017-0003.

Xu, G. Z., Li, Y. F., Wang, M. D., & Cao, D. Y. (2017). Complementary and alternative interventions for fatigue management after traumatic brain injury: A systematic review. *Therapeutic Advances in Neurological Disorders*, *10*(5), 229–239. Available from https://doi.org/10.1177/1756285616682675.

Yaeger, K., Alhilali, L., & Fakhran, S. (2014). Evaluation of tentorial length and angle in sleep-wake disturbances after mild traumatic brain injury. *AJR. American Journal of Roentgenology*, *202*(3), 614–618. Available from https://doi.org/10.2214/AJR.13.11091. Retrieved from <http://www.ncbi.nlm.nih.gov/pubmed/24555599>.

Zasler, N., Katz, D., & Zafonte, R. (2012). *Brain injury medicine: Principles and practice* (2nd ed.). New York: Demos Medical.

Ziino, C., & Ponsford, J. (2005). Measurement and prediction of subjective fatigue following traumatic brain injury. *Journal of the International Neuropsychological Society*, *11*(4), 416–425. Available from https://doi.org/10.1017/S1355617705050472. Retrieved from <http://www.ncbi.nlm.nih.gov/entrez/query.fcgi?cmd = Retrieve&db = PubMed&dopt = Citation&list_uids = 16209422>.

Ziino, C., & Ponsford, J. (2006). Vigilance and fatigue following traumatic brain injury. *Journal of the International Neuropsychological Society*, *12*(1), 100–110. Available from https://doi.org/10.1017/S1355617706060139. Retrieved from <http://www.ncbi.nlm.nih.gov/entrez/query.fcgi?cmd = Retrieve&db = PubMed&dopt = Citation&list_uids = 16433949>.

Zollman, F. S., Larson, E. B., Wasek-Throm, L. K., Cyborski, C. M., & Bode, R. K. (2012). Acupuncture for treatment of insomnia in patients with traumatic brain injury: A pilot intervention study. *Journal of Head Trauma Rehabilitation*, *27*, 135–142.

2

Assessment of Insomnia and Fatigue Following Traumatic Brain Injury

ASSESSMENT: A DYNAMIC PROCESS

An exhaustive assessment using a variety of tools will help the clinician grasp the predisposing, precipitating, and perpetuating factors underpinning the issues of insomnia or fatigue after traumatic brain injury (TBI). This comprehension is essential to guide the implementation of the various cognitive-behavioral intervention strategies. Although assessment and intervention are often conceptualized as two consecutive, distinct phases, they can be implemented in a much more dynamic way. Assessment usually takes place first, but it can be spread over a number of sessions and continue throughout the intervention phase. Conversely, some level of intervention can start early on in the process, if, for example, a specific treatment target is identified soon during assessment and can rapidly be acted upon (e.g., sleep hygiene change, irregular sleep schedule).

Several types of data collection can be combined when conducting a thorough assessment of insomnia and/or fatigue in the context of TBI. *Discrete assessment* is the most common form, involving the documentation of the patient's current state of difficulties and associated factors, using an interview or questionnaires. The latter are usually completed by the patient but can also be complemented by the perspective of a significant other. *Retrospective assessment* can be very helpful to characterize the evolution and antecedents of current difficulties, and putting these into the context of the history before and since the accident. Retrospective questions can be included in interviews and questionnaires but should also be interpreted in the light of potential biases such as a recall bias (having difficulty recalling the past) as well as a "good old days" bias where the patient may underestimate preinjury occasional issues with sleep or fatigue, or overestimate energy levels or sleep quality (SQ). Consultation of the patient's medical records and other key persons (e.g., significant others, treating clinicians) can provide invaluable information to complement the retrospective information. Finally, *prospective assessment* is used to gather data on sleep or energy patterns (e.g., within-day and between-day fluctuations) and also to monitor progress throughout the assessment and intervention phases. Daily self-monitoring tools (e.g., sleep or energy diaries) completed by the patient are typically used for prospective assessment and may be used as soon as the patient is able to complete them. In the acute phase postinjury, or with patients with significant cognitive impairments, actigraphy or observation logs, filled out by a family member or friend, or by attending medical personnel, may be alternatives for prospective assessment if self-monitoring is not feasible.

WHAT TO ASSESS

History, Nature, and Manifestations of Insomnia and Fatigue Symptoms Since the Injury

Assessment primarily focuses on the nature, severity, frequency, and fluctuations of the symptoms. To obtain a representative portrait, patients can be asked to refer to the past month when describing their symptoms (unless there was a significant change affecting sleep or energy in this period). A careful evaluation of the history of symptoms is warranted, notably to determine whether some insomnia or fatigue symptoms were present before the brain injury, and to document changes observed since the TBI (i.e., changes in the nature, frequency, and severity of symptoms), and try to pinpoint potentially aggravating factors. The clinician may also want to obtain a sense of the evolution of sleep/wake issues with different phases postinjury: during the acute or hospitalization phase, the weeks after returning home, when trying to return to work or to reintegrate other social roles, for example, and to evaluate whether the sleep or fatigue is persistent, episodic, gradually worsening, or gradually improving.

Impact of Insomnia and Fatigue Symptoms on Evolution of Brain Injury Condition/Adaptation

Insomnia is considered a 24-hour disorder, with both difficulty sleeping at night and difficulty functioning during the day. As such, it is essential to investigate both the nocturnal manifestations and the perceived daytime consequences of insomnia. The same also applies to fatigue, which can have a pervasive impact on several aspects of daily life, including the sleep—wake cycle. The following domains of functioning should be assessed, and patients can be asked to estimate if the contribution of sleep difficulties or fatigue in their functional impairments linked to TBI or not:

- Fatigue (when assessing insomnia consequences): tiredness, weariness
- Sleep difficulties (when assessing fatigue consequences): insomnia (initial, middle, late), hypersomnia, napping habits
- Daytime sleepiness: sleep propensity, drowsiness, lapses in vigilance
- Cognitive difficulties: exacerbation of memory, attention, and concentration problems
- Psychological distress: worrying or preoccupation related to insomnia or fatigue, about the impact of poor sleep on brain recovery, or mood disturbances such as marked discouragement, sadness, or irritability
- Impacts on motivation and initiative
- Physical symptoms: exacerbation of pain (related to the injury or not) and symptoms such as headaches and migraines, muscle tension, gastrointestinal problems
- Family and social life: avoidance of activities or commitments, behaviors and feelings during activities or commitments (e.g., more withdrawn during social gatherings, less enjoyment), potential reinforcement of illness behaviors by the entourage (e.g., significant others indefinitely taking up roles of the injured person to let them sleep or rest)

Habitual Sleep—Wake Schedule

A precise documentation of the person's typical sleep—wake cycle is important, including habitual bedtime and rising time, and night-to-night and weekdays-to-weekends variability. Regarding daytime napping, it is useful to gather information on the frequency, duration, timing, environment (i.e., in the bed or elsewhere), and amount of sleep obtained during daytime naps, both planned and unplanned (e.g., dozing off during a bus ride). The clinician should strive to understand if daytime and nighttime sleep habits have changed significantly from before the accident. In order to get a better understanding of the patient's typical schedule, questions can be asked about habitual activities (e.g., housework, social activities, sport/leisure activities, work or class schedules). This should be done tactfully and keeping in mind that the person may not have yet reintegrated certain preinjury roles because of injury-related limitations.

Medications and Treatments

Asking about past experiences with either medication or nonpharmacological interventions to manage sleep or fatigue difficulties is useful. In addition, it is essential to obtain a clear portrait of medications taken, to be aware of potential interactions between medications, and to keep in mind other medical conditions (e.g., orthopedic injuries causing pain) or psychiatric disorders (e.g., depression, anxiety, substance abuse), which may be contributing to sleep or fatigue issues. Indeed, several medications administered for treating various issues linked to the injury (e.g., analgesics, anticonvulsants, antidepressants, myorelaxants, corticosteroids) may influence daytime functioning or the quality, quantity, or structure of sleep depending on the pharmacokinetics of these compounds, their timing and dosage. Effective liaison with physicians prescribing medications either for sleep, vigilance, pain, mood, or other issues is essential to implement a careful evaluation and monitoring of the potential side effects and interactions of medications and to avoid effects on daytime alertness or other undesirable effects.

Lifestyle and Environmental Factors

Use of caffeine, nicotine, alcohol, and recreational drugs must be carefully documented. Substance use (e.g., alcohol, cannabis), which is quite common in TBI and other patient populations, is known to exacerbate fatigue or insomnia symptoms. Some persons may also use over-the-counter medications or substances specifically to manage their sleep or fatigue-related symptoms. Exercise habits, or lack of, should also be documented to determine if integrating regular exercise could increase energy levels or improve sleep or to pinpoint whether the timing of physical activities (e.g., vigorous activity too close to bedtime) may be influencing sleep. Finally, other environmental factors to consider include the sleep environment (e.g., bed and bedroom comfortable and quiet), and the exposure to natural and artificial light.

Screening for Other Sleep Disorders

It is important to question the patient and if possible a significant other about potential symptoms of other sleep disorders. Indeed, besides insomnia, sleep-disordered breathing disorders, narcolepsy, posttraumatic hypersomnia, and circadian rhythm sleep disorders are also observed following TBI more frequently than in the general population. Parasomnias and restless leg syndrome may also be present, but these disorders have not been specifically associated with TBI. Other sleep disorders may be comorbid with insomnia, and as such, failing to identify a comorbid sleep disorder can be detrimental to the outcome of insomnia treatment.

Investigate the following symptoms to rule out other sleep-related disorders:

Sleep apnea	Loud snoring, noticeable pauses of breath during the night, waking up choking, daytime sleepiness, headaches in the morning, dry mouth
Restless legs	Inability to keep legs still, aching or crawling feelings in the legs (during the night but also potentially during the day)
Periodic leg movements	Leg twitches, jerks, or cramps during the night
Parasomnias	Nightmare and sleep terrors, sleepwalking
Narcolepsy	Sleep attacks during the day, sensation of paralysis, hypnagogic hallucinations, cataplexy
Gastrointestinal condition	Heartburn, reflux, sour taste in the mouth

Screening for Psychopathology

Although fatigue and insomnia may be considered as stand-alone issues, these may also have developed or be exacerbated in the context of psychopathology. It is essential to screen for psychiatric disorders and refer for further evaluation if necessary. Indeed, up to 75% of persons who have suffered from TBI will present a psychiatric disorder in the first 5 years postinjury. Major depression and anxiety disorders are the most frequent diagnoses, and comorbidity between several psychiatric disorders is also very frequent. Having suffered a psychiatric disorder before the injury puts the individual at significantly greater risk of suffering from psychopathology postinjury.

TYPES OF ASSESSMENT

Clinical Interviews

An in-depth clinical interview will allow thorough documentation of the evolution, current severity, and potential causes of sleep/fatigue complaints. Ideally this interview would be complemented by information provided by a significant other living with the patient.

Post–Traumatic Brain Injury Insomnia Interview

For insomnia, we propose in this manual a semistructured interview canvas entitled *The Clinical Interview on Insomnia Following Traumatic Brain Injury*. This interview was adapted from the Insomnia Interview Schedule developed by Morin (1993). The latter interview was designed to assess insomnia but can also be used to gather information regarding other sleep–wake disturbances that may be present. It has been used extensively in clinical research to provide a guide to diagnosing insomnia and to facilitate the planning of treatment. It has previously been adapted to describe insomnia in different clinical populations presenting comorbid conditions such as cancer (Savard, Simard, Ivers, & Morin, 2005) and TBI (Ouellet, Beaulieu-Bonneau, & Morin, 2012).

The *Clinical Interview on Insomnia Following Traumatic Brain Injury* covers the following topics:

- The evolution and history of the sleep problem (onset, duration, evolution, and variations through time and in relation with the injury)
- Documentation of habitual sleep–wake schedule (initial bedtime, final arising time) including potential changes during weekends (or days where routines are different)
- Estimates of sleep onset latency (e.g., an estimate of the average number of minutes taken to fall asleep), typical number and duration of awakenings during the night, estimate of average total sleep time (TST)
- The nature of the sleep–wake complaint (problems falling asleep, difficulty remaining asleep, waking up too early in the morning, unusual experiences during sleep, daytime sleepiness)
- Daytime consequences of sleep problems (e.g., alterations of mood, fatigue, sleepiness, social issues and difficulty with concentration, memory or other cognitive impairment)
- Environmental factors (e.g., habitual levels of light and noise, room temperature, comfort-related issues)
- Use of different medications

- Factors linked to sleep hygiene (e.g., caffeine intake, use of nicotine, alcohol, or other drugs, physical exercise habits)
- Napping habits
- Snoring, interruptions in breathing
- Unusual events occurring at sleep onset or during the night (e.g., sleep terrors, cataplexy, hypnagogic hallucinations, paralysis, limb movements)
- Medical history (e.g., pain, anemia, hyperthyroidism)
- Questions to complete a functional analysis including antecedents, consequences, potential secondary gains

An abridged version is also provided if insomnia needs to be assessed more rapidly or if it is viewed as secondary compared to fatigue or another condition.

Post–Traumatic Brain Injury Fatigue Interview

For fatigue, we have developed the *Clinical Interview on Fatigue Following Traumatic Brain Injury*, also inspired from the Insomnia Interview Schedule proposed by Morin (1993). It covers the following topics:

- Documentation of current fatigue/energy levels and evolution since the injury
- Comparison of fatigue/energy levels before the injury
- Rest and nap-taking habits including timing and frequency of daytime sleep
- Consequences of fatigue (e.g., daily routine, mood, mental capacities, social/leisure/familial life, occupation)
- Potential causes of fatigue (e.g., anxiety, depressed mood, substance use, pain, medical problems, use of medication, physical inactivity)
- Current strategies to manage fatigue (e.g., naps, rest, reduction of activities)
- Impact of fatigue on significant others
- Exploration of activities reduced because of fatigue

Diaries

Daily self-monitoring instruments, or diaries, are particularly useful tools to assess insomnia (with a sleep diary) or fatigue (with an energy/ activity diary). They can be used both in the assessment phase and in the intervention phase. Completing such self-monitoring tools yields the benefits of giving clients an active role and restoring a certain sense of control in the management of their sleep or energy. Early in the assessment process, a sleep or energy diary completed every day for 1 or 2 weeks can provide a good portrait of the nature, severity, and fluctuations of the patient's difficulties. For patients with adequate introspection, filling out a diary allows them to better understand their sleep or energy patterns. Diaries can also help to identify intervention targets by revealing issues such as detrimental habits for sleep or fatigue, less-than-optimal planning or management of activities, or a clearly irregular sleep—wake schedule. When used over a longer period of time (a few weeks or months during treatment for example), the diary will allow for the application of therapeutic recommendations and the measurement of intervention effects. It can also provide precious information on adherence to treatment recommendations. In addition to blank sleep and energy diaries, this manual also provides detailed instructions on how to fill out the diaries (including examples) and recommendations on how to use and interpret data derived from sleep and energy diaries (see Part II, Chapters 4 and 5).

Sleep Diary

Several models of sleep diaries are available, including the consensus sleep diary, developed by a group of sleep experts (Carney et al., 2012). This book contains two sleep diaries: a complete 11-question version similar to the consensus sleep diary and an abridged 4-question version. The *full version* includes questions on (1) moment and duration of naps in the previous day, (2) bedtime, (3) time when started trying to fall asleep (lights-off time), (4) time taken to fall asleep, (5) number of nighttime awakenings, (6) total duration of nighttime awakenings, (7) number of times when got out of bed during the night, (8) time of final awakening (after which there was no further sleep), (9) rising time, (10) SQ rating (from 1 = very bad to 5 = very good), and (11) use of sleep aid the previous night (i.e., prescribed medications, over-the-counter or natural products, alcohol, or soft drugs). The *abridged version* of the sleep diary contains only four questions (bedtime, time taken to fall asleep, total time spent awake for all awakenings, rising time). This version could be used with patients with whom the use of the full version is not ideal, for example, because of impaired cognitive functions or limited motivation. Sleep diaries should ideally be completed within 1 hour of getting out of bed in the morning to reduce recall bias and create a self-monitoring habit. Some patients feel they need to be very precise when filling out the sleep diary. To reduce undue pressure, patients are usually instructed *not* to monitor the clock during the night to fill out the diary but rather to simply provide their best estimates. Indeed, it has been observed that monitoring the clock during the night to provide precise answers can lead to arousal and worsen insomnia symptoms.

Several key sleep parameters can be derived from the sleep diary. First, the following variables can be directly obtained, usually averaged over a period of at least 1 week (we refer here to the full version): sleep onset latency (SOL; question 4), number of awakenings (question 5), wake after sleep onset (WASO; question 6), early morning awakening (EMA; time elapsed in minutes between time of final awakening, question 8, and rising time, question 9), and SQ (question 10). Then, the following variables can be calculated: *total time in bed* (TIB; obtained by calculating the time elapsed in minutes between the time when started trying to fall asleep, question 3, and rising time, question 9); *total wake time* (TWT; obtained by the summation of SOL, WASO, and EMA); TST (obtained by subtracting TWT from TIB); and *sleep efficiency* (SE; obtained by dividing TST by TIB, and multiplying the result by 100). A SE of 85%–90% or above is considered to be good according to most sleep experts, while a SE under this threshold is usually associated with restless, interrupted, and unsatisfying sleep. It is noteworthy that the main goal of restriction of TIB, one of the main behavioral components of cognitive-behavioral therapy for insomnia, is not to increase TST, but to improve SE.

Energy/Activity Diary

Compared to the sleep diary, there is less standardization for the content of an energy or fatigue diary. The main objectives are to document the patterns of energy levels (e.g., fluctuations within a day, fluctuations from one day to another), identify time periods when energy is lower and others when energy is higher, and, perhaps most importantly, examine the relationships between energy levels and activities, behaviors, and emotions. Researchers and clinicians working with patients with TBI collaboratively designed the 7-day energy diary provided in this book. The energy diary includes information about bedtime and rising time (important if sleep is not otherwise monitored), and each day is separated into five time periods (upon waking, morning, afternoon, dinnertime, evening) for which respondents have to rate their level of fatigue/energy with a "fatigue barometer" (a simple Likert scale from 1 to 5 where 1 = no fatigue, maximal energy; 5 = maximal fatigue, no energy), and record what they were doing, including inactivity periods (e.g., activities, meals, naps) or how they were feeling (e.g., emotions) at the time of their rating. As for the sleep diary, fatigue ratings for each period of the day can be averaged over 1 week to obtain a more global picture of fatigue levels. It is also essential to analyze the relationship between fatigue and activities or emotions, for instance, by identifying the activities associated with minimal fatigue and those associated with maximal fatigue. The number and diversity of the activities recorded are also important to consider. By taking the time to collaboratively analyze the energy/activity diary at every session with the patient, the clinician can identify intervention targets (e.g., modifying timing or planning of activities) and foster long-term self-management skills on the part of the patient.

Questionnaires

Research on insomnia and fatigue following TBI largely uses a variety of self-report questionnaires. In the vast majority of cases, even in cases of severe TBI, the presence of cognitive deficits generally does not preclude the use of such self-report instruments. It is however possible that in some cases self-reported data may not be reliable because of severe cognitive or language issues or significantly impaired self-awareness. The Insomnia Severity Index (ISI) (Morin, 1993) and the Pittsburgh Sleep Quality Index (PSQI) (Buysse, Reynolds, Monk, Berman, & Kupfer, 1989) are instruments which have been validated and used in samples of persons with TBI (Fichtenberg, Putnam, Mann, Zafonte, & Millard, 2001; Kaufmann et al., 2017; Lequerica et al., 2014). The ISI is included in the present manual. The PSQI is not specific to insomnia per se but measures sleep quality in general. It is available for clinical practice and clinical research (consult: https://eprovide.mapi-trust.org). Although still at the stage of validation, the Sleep and Concussion Questionnaire (Wiseman-Hakes & Ouellet, 2016; available in the Ontario Neurotrauma Foundation Guideline for Concussion/Mild Traumatic Brain Injury & Persistent Symptoms; https://braininjuryguidelines.org/concussion) was developed to identify and quantify changes in sleep after a concussion or other brain injury and to monitor these changes over time.

Subjective self-report instruments are also very useful to assess fatigue in TBI survivors. A variety of instruments exist including the Fatigue Impact Scale (Fisk et al., 1994), the Fatigue Severity Scale (Krupp, LaRocca, Muir-Nash, & Steinberg, 1989), the Global Fatigue Index (Belza, Henke, Yelin, Epstein, & Gilliss, 1993), and the Multidimensional Fatigue Inventory (MFI; Smets et al., 1995), although these were not devised or validated specifically for a brain-injured population. Borgaro, Gierok, Caples, and Kwasnica (2004) developed a short instrument specifically for the TBI population: the *Barrow Neurological Institute Fatigue Scale*. While most measures are one-dimensional scales (measure a general feeling of fatigue), fatigue is generally considered to be a multidimensional phenomenon. The MFI is one instrument exploring various potential facets of fatigue. It includes five dimensions of fatigue: general fatigue, physical fatigue, mental fatigue, impact of fatigue on motivation, and impact of fatigue on reduction of activities. This manual includes the MFI and the Fatigue Severity Scale.

To punctually assess fatigue (at one moment in time), simple numerical (e.g., rating fatigue on a scale from 1 to 10) or visual analog scales can be used. As a more visual tool, this manual also proposes a simple fatigue barometer (using a battery metaphor for energy reserve) where the patient simply evaluates his/her fatigue on a scale from 1 to 5. It is particularly useful during intervention to develop awareness of fatigue/ energy levels especially when patients start experimenting with modifications to habits and/or activities.

Objective Measures

Patients with TBI may sometimes be referred for a sleep study that involves nighttime or daytime polysomnography (PSG). An insomnia diagnosis does not require nighttime PSG however. Nighttime PSG may be considered if other sleep disorders need to be ruled out such as obstructive sleep apnea, central sleep apnea, upper airway resistance syndrome, nocturnal seizures (Kushida et al., 2005). Access to PSG is often limited however, since it requires highly specialized facilities (when conducted in a laboratory), equipment, and personnel.

Nighttime Polysomnography

Nighttime PSG provides an objective measure of sleep and can be conducted either in a sleep laboratory or at home with ambulatory equipment (the latter having the advantage of measuring sleep in a more naturalistic setting but providing less control over potential artifacts). Nighttime PSG will usually monitor various parameters of brain activity, as well as breathing and limb movements. PSG provides a comprehensive documentation of sleep parameters such as exact SOL, time to onset of different sleep stages, time spent in the different sleep stages, time spent awake after sleep onset, TST, and SE. A hypnogram (graph of sleep parameters) is usually produced. The sleep study generally involves at least one night in a specialized laboratory, although more nights are needed to provide a more ecologically valid assessment, especially when performed in a laboratory to allow patients to get adapted to this unfamiliar environment and equipment. Trained technicians process PSG data according to standardized criteria. A standard PSG montage usually includes electroencephalographic (brain activity), electrooculographic (eye movements), and electromyographic (muscle movements) recordings. Additional measures may also be administered, such as airflow, heart rate, blood oxygenation, and muscle movements, monitored through electrocardiograms, thoracic or abdominal straps, nasal sensors of airflow, electrodes on leg muscles (anterior tibialis), or oxymeters placed on the fingertip (Besset, 2003).

Daytime Polysomnography

Daytime PSG may be considered if disorders linked to excessive daytime sleepiness are suspected. The Multiple Sleep Latency Test consists in monitoring SOL during four or five nap opportunities of 20 minutes, each spaced at 2-hour intervals. Excessive sleepiness is defined as a mean SOL of less than 5 minutes (Mahowald & Mahowald, 1996). This test may be useful in diagnosing narcolepsy. The Maintenance of Wakefulness Test is another daytime PSG test of sleepiness where patients are instructed to stay awake during several 40-minute periods. Persons who fall asleep in less than 5 minutes during the nap opportunities are considered to have excessive daytime sleepiness. This test may be particularly relevant to inform whether the person can stay awake, especially in patients for whom fluctuations in vigilance or cognitive function seem to be an important issue post-TBI (Arand et al., 2005; Castriotta et al., 2009).

Actigraphy

An actigraph may be considered as a lower cost alternative to PSG. It can also be useful to appreciate the distribution of activity/inactivity levels over the 24-hour period. An actigraph is usually a small watch-like device that continuously records activity data (and sometimes also luminosity) over several days regarding motor activity over several days (Ancoli-Israel & Ayalon, 2006). Actigraphs have been used in several studies following brain injury, although caution is in order if the patient presents spasticity, paresis, agitation, or impulsivity. Adaptations such as placing the device on the least affected limb if motor impairments are present may be considered (Muller, Czymmek, Thone-Otto, & Von Cramon, 2006; Zollman, Cyborski, & Duraski, 2010).

ASSESSING THE PATIENTS' READINESS FOR INTERVENTION

Before beginning interventions for post-TBI insomnia or fatigue, it is important to consider whether the patient is likely to be able to benefit from the strategies proposed in this manual: at a minimum, the patient should show some capacity for introspection, adequate comprehension, and openness to learning to self-manage energy or sleep habits. Furthermore, for therapy to be successful, a relatively high level of commitment to adhering to treatment recommendations is necessary. Patients with very limited self-awareness or with very severe behavioral or cognitive issues might be less able to engage in such an intervention. In these cases, modifications to the environment or focusing on key sleep hygiene factors (e.g., caffeine/nicotine intake) or attempting to regularize the sleep/wake schedule may be the only feasible nonpharmacological options. It is important to note that self-awareness and behavioral and cognitive issues may evolve favorably, and as such, readiness for intervention can be evaluated at different time points. By taking into consideration the expertise of clinicians developed over the years (e.g., occupational therapists, neuropsychologists) working in post-TBI rehabilitation (both inpatient and outpatient contexts), Cantin, Ouellet, Turcotte, Lessard, Potvin, Boutin, and Duchesneau (2014) have identified key patient characteristics can help the clinician to gauge readiness for intervention.

Indicators of better patient receptiveness and greater potential for success	Indicators of more limited patient receptiveness and lower potential for success
• Shows adequate self-awareness • Has at least a minimal capacity for introspection • Shows motivation for improving his or her personal functioning • Takes advantage of experience to make subsequent adjustments • Can recognize and respect his or her strengths or limitations • Has sufficient adaptive capabilities • Accepts that changes may take time • Enjoys the active support of family/friends	• Is not interested in analyzing his or her personal functioning • Shows significant cognitive rigidity • Does not want to change habits • Demonstrates significant apathy • Considers other issues as more important compared to fatigue or insomnia • Is careless, indifferent, or very passive • Has family/friends who continually compensate for his or her difficulties or fatigue

Adapted with permission of the authors from Cantin, J. F., Ouellet, M.-C., Turcotte, N., Lessard, J., Potvin, I., Boutin, N., & Duchesneau, G. (2014). Guide de l'énergie: vers une meilleure gestion de la fatigue. Québec: Institut de réadaptation en déficience physique de Québec.

Assessment Tools Suggested in This Manual

	Insomnia	Fatigue
Semistructured interviews	• Clinical interview on insomnia (full and abridged versions)	• Clinical interview on fatigue
Self-monitoring tools	• Sleep diary (full and abridged versions)	• Energy/Activity diary
Questionnaires	• Insomnia Severity Index • Beliefs and attitudes about sleep scale	• Multidimensional sleep inventory • Fatigue Severity Scale • Fatigue numerical rating scale • Fatigue barometer

Note: The use of different types of tools is recommended for a flexible and complete assessment.

References

Ancoli-Israel, S., & Ayalon, L. (2006). Diagnosis and treatment of sleep disorders in older adults. *American Journal of Geriatric Psychiatry*, *14*(2), 95−103. Available from https://doi.org/10.1097/01.JGP.0000196627.12010.d1. Retrieved from <http://www.ncbi.nlm.nih.gov/entrez/query.fcgi?cmd = Retrieve&db = PubMed&dopt = Citation&list_uids = 16473973>.

Arand, D., Bonnet, M., Hurwitz, T., Mitler, M., Rosa, R., & Sangal, R. B. (2005). The clinical use of the MSLT and MWT. *Sleep*, *28*(1), 123−144. Retrieved from <http://www.ncbi.nlm.nih.gov/entrez/query.fcgi?cmd = Retrieve&db = PubMed&dopt = Citation&list_uids = 15700728>.

Belza, B. L., Henke, C. J., Yelin, E. H., Epstein, W. V., & Gilliss, C. L. (1993). Correlates of fatigue in older adults with rheumatoid arthritis. *Nursing Research*, *42*(2), 93−99.

Besset, A. (2003). Polysomnography. In M. Billiard (Ed.), *Sleep: Physiology, investigations and medicine* (pp. 127−138). New York: Plenum Publishers.

Borgaro, S. R., Gierok, S., Caples, H., & Kwasnica, C. (2004). Fatigue after brain injury: Initial reliability study of the BNI Fatigue Scale. *Brain Injury*, *18*(7), 685−690. Available from https://doi.org/10.1080/02699050310001646080. Retrieved from <http://www.ncbi.nlm.nih.gov/entrez/query.fcgi?cmd = Retrieve&db = PubMed&dopt = Citation&list_uids = 15204329>.

Buysse, D. J., Reynolds, C. F., 3rd, Monk, T. H., Berman, S. R., & Kupfer, D. J. (1989). The Pittsburgh Sleep Quality Index: A new instrument for psychiatric practice and research. *Psychiatry Research*, *28*(2), 193−213. Retrieved from <http://www.ncbi.nlm.nih.gov/entrez/query.fcgi?cmd = Retrieve&db = PubMed&dopt = Citation&list_uids = 2748771>.

Cantin, J. F., Ouellet, M.-C., Turcotte, N., Lessard, J., Potvin, I., Boutin, N., & Duchesneau, G. (2014). *Guide de l'énergie: vers une meilleure gestion de la fatigue*. Québec: Institut de réadaptation en déficience physique de Québec.

Carney, C. E., Buysse, D. J., Ancoli-Israel, S., Edinger, J. D., Krystal, A. D., Lichstein, K. L., & Morin, C. M. (2012). The consensus sleep diary: Standardizing prospective sleep self-monitoring. *Sleep*, *35*(2), 287−302. Available from https://doi.org/10.5665/sleep.1642.

Castriotta, R. J., Atanasov, S., Wilde, M. C., Masel, B. E., Lai, J. M., & Kuna, S. T. (2009). Treatment of sleep disorders after traumatic brain injury. *Journal of Clinical Sleep Medicine: JCSM: Official Publication of the American Academy of Sleep Medicine, 5*(2), 137–144.

Fichtenberg, N. L., Putnam, S. H., Mann, N. R., Zafonte, R. D., & Millard, A. E. (2001). Insomnia screening in postacute traumatic brain injury: Utility and validity of the Pittsburgh Sleep Quality Index. *American Journal of Physical Medicine & Rehabilitation, 80* (5), 339–345. Retrieved from <http://www.ncbi.nlm.nih.gov/pubmed/11327555>.

Fisk, J. D., Ritvo, P. G., Ross, L., Haase, D. A., Marrie, T. J., & Schlech, W. F. (1994). Measuring the functional impact of fatigue: Initial validation of the Fatigue Impact Scale. *Clinical Infectious Diseases, 18*(Suppl. 1), S79–83. Retrieved from <http://www. ncbi.nlm.nih.gov/entrez/query.fcgi?cmd = Retrieve&db = PubMed&dopt = Citation &list_uids = 8148458>.

Kaufmann, C. N., Orff, H. J., Moore, R. C., Delano-Wood, L., Depp, C. A., & Schiehser, D. M. (2017). Psychometric characteristics of the Insomnia Severity Index in veterans with history of traumatic brain injury. *Behavioral Sleep Medicine*, 1–9. Available from https://doi.org/10.1080/15402002.2016.1266490.

Krupp, L. B., LaRocca, N. G., Muir-Nash, J., & Steinberg, A. D. (1989). The Fatigue Severity Scale. Application to patients with multiple sclerosis and systemic lupus erythematosus. *Archives of Neurology, 46*(10), 1121–1123. Retrieved from <http://www.ncbi.nlm. nih.gov/entrez/query.fcgi?cmd = Retrieve&db = PubMed&dopt = Citation&list_uids = 2803071>.

Kushida, C. A., Littner, M. R., Morgenthaler, T., Alessi, C. A., Bailey, D., Coleman, J., Jr., ... Wise, M. (2005). Practice parameters for the indications for polysomnography and related procedures: An update for 2005. *Sleep, 28*(4), 499–521.

Lequerica, A., Chiaravalloti, N., Cantor, J., Dijkers, M., Wright, J., Kolakowsky-Hayner, S. A., ... Bell, K. (2014). The factor structure of the Pittsburgh Sleep Quality Index in persons with traumatic brain injury. A NIDRR TBI model systems module study. *NeuroRehabilitation, 35*(3), 485–492. Available from https://doi.org/10.3233/nre-141141.

Mahowald, M., & Mahowald, M. (1996). Sleep disorders. In M. Rizzo, & D. Tranel (Eds.), *Head injury and postconcussive syndrome* (pp. 285–304). New York: Churchill Livingstone.

Morin, C. (1993). *Insomnia: Psychological assessment and management.* New York: Guilford.

Muller, U., Czymmek, J., Thone-Otto, A., & Von Cramon, D. Y. (2006). Reduced daytime activity in patients with acquired brain damage and apathy: A study with ambulatory actigraphy. *Brain Injury, 20*(2), 157–160.

Ouellet, M. C., Beaulieu-Bonneau, S., & Morin, C. M. (2012). Sleep-wake disturbances. In N. Zasler, D. Katz, & R. Zafonte (Eds.), *Brain injury medicine: Principles and practice* (2nd ed., pp. 707–725). Boston, MA: Demos Medical Publishing.

Savard, J., Simard, S., Ivers, H., & Morin, C. M. (2005). Randomized study on the efficacy of cognitive-behavioral therapy for insomnia secondary to breast cancer, Part I: Sleep and psychological effects. *Journal of Clinical Oncology, 23*(25), 6083–6096. Retrieved from <http://www.ncbi.nlm.nih.gov/entrez/query.fcgi?cmd = Retrieve&db = PubMed&dopt = Citation&list_uids = 16135475>.

Smets, E. M., Garssen, B., Bonke, B., & De Haes, J. C. (1995). The Multidimensional Fatigue Inventory (MFI) psychometric qualities of an instrument to assess fatigue. *Journal of Psychosomatic Research, 39*(3), 315–325. Retrieved from <http://www.ncbi.nlm.nih. gov/entrez/query.fcgi?cmd = Retrieve&db = PubMed&dopt = Citation&list_uids = 7636775>.

Zollman, F. S., Cyborski, C., & Duraski, S. A. (2010). Actigraphy for assessment of sleep in traumatic brain injury: Case series, review of the literature and proposed criteria for use. *Brain Injury, 24*(5), 748–754.

3

CBT Interventions for Insomnia and Fatigue in the Context of TBI: Rationale, Adaptations, and Clinical Challenges

This chapter presents each treatment component proposed in this manual. Several components pertain to both post−traumatic brain injury (TBI) insomnia and fatigue, while others are used more specifically in the context of either insomnia or fatigue. For each component, we briefly expose the rationale and provide guidelines for implementation. The information in this chapter can be complemented with the tools presented in Chapters 6 and 7, which will guide the implementation of each treatment component. The present chapter also presents different clinical challenges that are specific to implementing cognitive−behavioral therapy (CBT) for insomnia and fatigue in the TBI population. Indeed, administering CBT for insomnia in the context of TBI requires certain adaptations to account for potential issues linked to the injury such as cognitive issues, physical limitations, behavioral particularities, or the presence of psychological comorbidities, which will be discussed.

GENERAL COGNITIVE−BEHAVIORAL THERAPY TREATMENT COMPONENTS

Fostering a Self-Management Approach

Rationale

Building a strong alliance and fostering active involvement on the part of the patient is essential from the beginning of a CBT intervention process for insomnia and fatigue. Indeed, because the proposed intervention strategies require substantial effort and commitment on the part of patients, collaboratively working toward goals is a key ingredient in intervention outcome. Rather than being overly directive, the clinician can rather strive to take on the role of a coach or guide. The self-management approach aims to empower patients with respect to their lifestyle habits, behaviors, attitudes, and thoughts, so that they can feel they are acquiring some control over their sleep or energy levels. CBT aims the acquisition of skills that will be used over the long term to manage fatigue and sleep difficulties. Because of the often chronic nature of insomnia and fatigue in patients with TBI, the clinician should reinforce the fact that CBT will help them to lower the impact of insomnia or fatigue on their activities and social roles, through different sleep and energy management strategies but is unlikely to completely eliminate these problems. Rather, the goal is to increase quality of life and social participation despite the presence of some sleep or fatigue issues. It is important for the clinician to take the necessary time to thoroughly present the rationale of the different intervention strategies (and to repeat these as needed), to foster collaboration toward common goals, and to take a step back when resistance is occurring.

Implementation

The following points can be discussed openly with patients at the beginning of the intervention as well as later moments during the intervention as needed.

Fostering Commitment and Effort

The clinician's role is to analyze the patient's situation and to suggest strategies in order to improve the patient's sleep and energy level. The majority of the therapeutic work, of course, is implemented by the patient in daily life. Ideally, the patient will demonstrate willingness to commit to practicing the strategies discussed in order to test their effectiveness. Several strategies involve changes in ingrained behavior or attitude, and consequently require time and constant effort on the part of the patient. Several weeks of steady application may be required before an improvement can be seen clearly. If issues with motivation are at hand, a motivational approach can be used, delaying the beginning of sleep or fatigue-targeted strategies or taking a pause during these, if needed. Motivational interviewing techniques which can be considered include expressing empathy about difficulty to adhere to recommendations, rolling with resistance, and exploring ways to enhance the patient's self-efficacy.

Keeping Realistic Goals

It is useful to ask the patient about his or her expectations with regards to improving sleep or energy level and to start by assessing collaboratively the realism of the patient's goals. For example, several individuals may want to go "back to normal" or will constantly compare their sleep or energy level to "before the accident." It is important to make sure that the patients' goals remain realistic given the injury incurred. Some patients may also hope that if they sleep better, their fatigue will disappear. Although post-TBI insomnia and fatigue interinfluence each other, they can also be independent problems (Ouellet & Morin, 2006). As such, improving sleep will not automatically mean that personal functioning during the day will improve to the same degree (e.g., in terms of fatigue and energy level), and vice versa. It can help to have a discussion about first lowering the impact of these problems on everyday functioning and quality of life. Patients can be encouraged to focus on recent progress instead of comparing themselves to "before" the injury, as this can foster a more encouraging perspective.

Adopting a Scientific Attitude

Throughout the intervention, clinicians will invite patients to perform behavioral experiments and to self-monitor what may happen when changes to habits, thoughts, or attitudes are introduced. This implies that the patient is open to these "experiments" and is willing to keep an open mind and stay aware during these changes. Fully explaining the rationale of the interventions, and verifying that both the patient and clinician are working collaboratively toward the same goal, will help the process. Clinicians may underline, for example, that it is preferable not to draw conclusions about the efficacy of intervention before having tested it thoroughly and observed objectively the effects, much as a scientist would do. It is also essential for patients to take the time to integrate treatment recommendations into their daily life, to try them out for a certain period of time (at least a few weeks) and to make some adaptations, if needed, before judging their effectiveness.

Establishing Effective Self-Monitoring

Rationale

Self-monitoring is the cornerstone of cognitive–behavioral interventions (Cohen, Edmunds, Brodman, Benjamin, & Kendall, 2013). It provides the patient a concrete tool to observe his or her own behaviors, thoughts, and overall habits, observations that can then be shared with the therapist during structured treatment, or used by the person after treatment to maintain treatment gains. Self-monitoring is routinely used in the assessment phases of CBT for insomnia and fatigue in clinical and research contexts: it also represents an active ingredient of therapy per se. Indeed, it contributes to the patients' sense of control over their behaviors or reactions and provides a way for patients to take emotional distance from the problems they face by adopting a "scientific" attitude. As such, self-monitoring contributes to prepare the patient to consider making changes to his or her habits. It also clearly gives the patient an active role in therapy from the start.

Specifically, in the context of *sleep* issues, self-monitoring first allows a documentation of sleep habits and behavior patterns which may contribute to insomnia, for example, by describing the severity and frequency of sleep difficulties, identifying circumstances and factors associated with a poor night of sleep, and thus identifying targets for treatment. A self-monitoring phase before initiating a specific treatment strategy will help provide greater perspective, by demonstrating that in spite of insomnia, there might exist periods where sleep is better. During the intervention for insomnia, self-monitoring will allow the patient to begin to implement self-management behaviors such as changing sleep-related habits and establishing a regular schedule. Progress may be evaluated with self-monitoring tools by logging carefully the progression of time spent awake, time spent sleeping, and sleep efficiency.

In the context of *fatigue*, self-monitoring not only allows a precise documentation of the severity of fatigue throughout a given day or week, but it can also reveal connections between activities and levels of fatigue. Self-monitoring can show, for example, marked periods of inactivity, or periods of overexertion followed by an increased need to rest. This information is also key to develop a balance between different types of activities (i.e., physical, productive, social, and leisure) and to identify how activities could be managed or planned differently, how some activities can be reintegrated, and how others can be increased or decreased. During intervention, self-monitoring is also an essential tool to help the patient recognize that some level of activity can be accomplished in spite of fatigue, albeit with some modifications of expectations, intensity, or duration. As such, self-monitoring may help the patient gradually modify negative perceptions about fatigue and his or her capacities and make a place for a more positive and motivating appraisal of his or her level of functioning.

Implementation

Patients with TBI may have more difficulty learning to use and fill out a sleep or energy/activity or fatigue diary if cognitive issues are present. It is important to establish an effective routine of self-monitoring before initiating treatment and to adapt the diary if the patient has problems filling it out properly. In the first weeks of self-monitoring with a sleep or energy/activity diary (at least 1–2 weeks), it is essential to closely monitor whether the patient understands and satisfactorily records information in the diary. Chapters 6 and 7 include Clinician Guides entitled "Establishing effective self-monitoring" containing different strategies to help establish and maintain the patient's self-monitoring habits and encourage adherence.

Sleep Diary

In this manual, we propose two versions of a sleep diary (a standard version with 11 questions and a simpler version that may be used if the standard version is too complex, for example, in the presence of more severe cognitive limitations). These can be reproduced on paper but any other alternatives to collect the same information can be considered. Indeed, the patient could also use an electronic device (e.g., computer, smartphone, and tablet) to monitor sleep, as long as it contains the same key information as in the proposed sleep diary. Any version of a sleep diary that contains the basic information in the abridged version is suitable to augment patient motivation. The information must at least allow the clinician, and eventually the patients themselves, to calculate sleep efficiency. Free applications for electronic devices exist and allow the self-monitoring of sleep but should be selected on the basis of simplicity of use and adequacy of information to reveal patterns of behavior. As such, the "good old" sheet of paper, word document, or excel spreadsheet is ideal as it allows the patient and clinician to have an overall view of a whole week of sleep–wake patterns.

Energy/Activity Diary

We propose an energy/activity diary that can be used flexibly to note down fatigue levels at different time point during the day (using a simple numerical scale), as well as activities, thoughts, and emotions. Ideally, patients will experiment with this diary long enough to reveal meaningful patterns between activities and energy levels (at least 1 or 2 weeks, and ideally throughout the intervention). Some patients might eventually want to use their own paper or electronic activity planner (or personal organizer, appointment planner). This can be encouraged, as it may be a sign that patients are getting well engaged with the intervention and integrating the recommendations. The clinician can oversee the change in self-monitoring tool over a few weeks, for example, by helping the patient to integrate a systematic scale to consistently charac-terize fatigue or energy (fatigue barometer, numerical or categorical scale) and making sure that the format of the diary or daily planner allows a global analysis of patterns of activity and rest.

COGNITIVE–BEHAVIORAL THERAPY COMPONENTS SPECIFICALLY FOR POST–TBI INSOMNIA

Psychoeducation About Normal Sleep, Sleep After Traumatic Brain Injury, and Insomnia

Rationale

Providing the patient with basic information about how sleep is affected by TBI, as well as information on normal sleep and the development of insomnia, will help support treatment. Indeed, this knowledge will allow the patient to better understand the potential multiple causes of sleep disturbances, will validate or normalize cer-tain subjective experiences, and will help identify factors over which he or she may have some control. Having a basic knowledge of sleep stages might help understand, for example, why some awakenings occur in the middle of the night, why sleeping seems lighter toward the end of the night, why lapses in vigilance and energy may occur in midafternoon, and why naps that are too long can affect the next night's sleep.

Implementation

Chapter 6 provides a series of Clinician Guides and tools to support psychoeducation on sleep in general, sleep after TBI, and insomnia. Some patients will be eager to acquire such knowledge and will be able to do so easily and on their own. Others will find the information too complex or academic; others will be interested but may forget the infor-mation or not refer to it. Considering the patient's level of education, lit-eracy and cognitive functioning, the clinician can choose to use these tools in part, in full or not at all depending on the cognitive limitations of the patients, their motivation to acquire more knowledge, and their reading skills. This psychoeducation component can help patients to realize that they have a control on certain factors that maintain insomnia over time and contribute to patient motivation and commitment. The visual elements (figures) may support some discussions about normal sleep or insomnia during sessions.

Sleep Hygiene Education

Rationale

Sleep hygiene education consists of providing the patient with knowledge concerning health-related habits that are known to have an impact on sleep including diet, exercise, use of alcohol, drugs, or medications use. It also includes information on which environmental factors (e.g., noise, light, temperature, and comfort) can also interfere with sleep. Although sleep hygiene education is largely used in medical practice, it is often insufficient to treat chronic insomnia (Morgenthaler et al., 2006).

Implementation

The evaluation may have pointed to certain life habits that are clearly linked to insomnia. Some changes to these habits can be more readily implemented by patients directly in the context of the intervention, such as the timing of exercise (not too close to bedtime), avoiding caffeine in the afternoon and evening, understanding the effects of alcohol on sleep onset and sleep quality. For life habits that are much more complex to change, such as substance use and dependence (e.g., smoking during the night), or changes in diet, motivational interviewing and/or referral to specialized programs or health professionals (e.g., nutritionist, exercise therapist, substance use program) might be necessary. Although the intervention for insomnia or fatigue can be initiated even in the presence of these problems or in parallel with other services, the outcomes may not be as positive if the life habits are clearly affecting sleep.

Restriction of Time in Bed: Limiting Time Spent in Bed to Actual Sleeping Time

Rationale

This treatment component was originally proposed by Spielman, Saskin, and Thorpy (1987) and has been shown to be a particularly effective therapeutic technique in CBT for insomnia (Miller et al., 2014). In our tools for patients, we have adapted the name of the intervention somewhat (Limiting time spent in bed to actual sleeping time) to reflect more closely what strategy the patient needs to put into place and to circumvent any resistance because the name of the intervention might appear counterintuitive. Persons suffering from insomnia tend to increase the time they spend in bed in the hope of obtaining more sleep or rest. In the short term, this strategy may seem to be useful, but if used on a long-term scale, it can lead to poor sleep because sleep is more fragmented. The aim of restriction of time in bed is thus to consolidate sleep on a shorter period. The intervention tends to create a state of mild sleep deprivation in the first few days or weeks that strengthens the homeostatic sleep drive that in turn helps reduce time to sleep onset and awakenings. This strategy also tends to lessen the patient's "performance" anxiety before bed; indeed, instead of focusing on trying to sleep as early as possible, the patient has to stay awake at least until the time prescribed by his or her sleep window. For example, for a sleep window where bedtime is postponed until midnight, this often has a paradoxical effect and changes the patient's focus of attention from "I must get to sleep by 11:00 p.m." to "what can I do to stay awake until the prescribed bedtime?" Caution is warranted since the implementation of this intervention component may produce daytime sleepiness and affect daytime vigilance or even reaction times. The sleep window should be of at least 5 hours, even for patients who report sleeping less than 5 hours.

Implementation

An initial sleep window is set so that time spent in bed corresponds to the actual sleep time (as calculated with at least 1 week of sleep diary data), thus producing mild sleep deprivation at the beginning of the intervention. Over time, and depending on the patient's progress (e.g., reduced time spent awake at night, increased sleep efficiency), the sleep window is gradually elongated throughout the treatment until an optimal sleep duration is attained. For example, for a person reporting spending an average of 8 hours in bed but who in fact sleeps 6 hours, the initial prescribed sleep window will be of 6 hours (i.e., 6 hours from bedtime to final arising time). A half hour can be added to this window (i.e., 6.5 hours in the case of the previous example) for slightly more flexibility, increased adherence if patients are more apprehensive of this therapy technique, or in cases of daytimes sleepiness. A whole week is spent using the prescribed sleep window, and self-monitoring is key. Indeed, the sleep diary data then allows the patient and clinician to collaboratively examine progress over the week with the prescribed sleep window; if sleep efficiency (total sleep time over time in bed $\times 100\%$) for that week has increased and now exceeds 85%, the sleep window may be increased by about 15–20 minutes for the next week. If, on the contrary, sleep efficiency is lower than 80%, the sleep window is decreased by 15–20 minutes. If sleep efficiency is between 80% and 85%, the same sleep window can be set for the next week. The sleep window can be adjusted by either postponing bedtime or advancing arising time, or both. Regardless of initial sleep duration, the sleep window should be no less than 5 hours per night in order to prevent daytime sleepiness. This is particularly important for persons who have jobs where lapses in vigilance may be dangerous, for example, persons operating machinery or motor vehicles. Adjustments to the sleep window are made every week until optimal or reasonable sleep duration is achieved. It is important to note that the optimal amount of sleep is not necessarily 8 hours for everyone. Often times, sleeping 6.5 or 7 hours with minimal interruptions is more restorative and satisfying than sleeping 8 hours with multiple and lengthy awakenings.

Notwithstanding the guidelines presented above to determine the ideal sleep window for optimal outcome, the sleep window should nonetheless be collaboratively agreed upon with the patient, taking into account the latter's willingness and perception of being able to adhere to the sleep window. A certain level of flexibility is warranted if the patient seems unsure of his or her capacity to adhere to the sleep window, while considering that a sleep window slightly too long may produce less optimal outcomes. Indeed, an approach that is too rigid may lead to poor adherence.

Adhering to the sleep window can be particularly challenging for patients who do not have a regular routine. For example, some persons may not be able to return to work for several months or even years following TBI and thus do not necessarily need to get up at a specific time every day. The clinician may need to explore different types of activities to determine what activity (or activities) could be planned into the patient's morning routine to help him or her rise and start being active at a regular and appropriate time. Planning pleasurable morning activities, in particular, can be useful to enhance motivation. Exploring what morning activities are pleasurable to the patient (e.g., cooking breakfast, preparing a hot beverage, reading or watching the news, taking a walk, taking care of indoor or outdoor plants, engaging in a gentle exercise routine) and focusing on how the sleep window can allow time for these activities may be useful.

In the evening, if staying up and awake until the prescribed bedtime is an issue, appropriate activities can also be explored and discussed with the patient. Building lists of activities that are pleasurable and appropriate in the evening and morning for this particular patient are useful. Consulting with an occupational therapist or with a leisure specialist is useful and important if the activities of the patient seem very limited.

Stimulus Control: Recreating a Time and Space for Sleep

Rationale

It is not uncommon for persons with insomnia to develop negative emotions and apprehensions close to bedtime, or even when entering their bedroom. Through a conditioning process, they may have come to associate specific environmental cues (bedroom environment) or temporal cues (nighttime) with the frustration of being unable to fall asleep or lying in bed for long periods of time trying to fall back asleep during the night. For good sleepers, presleep habits or rituals are usually associated with a relaxed state, and the temporal and environmental cues can, in fact, contribute to predispose the person favorably to sleep. For the person suffering from insomnia, these cues may have gradually become associated with activation, rumination, worrying, and being awake.

Stimulus control aims to reestablish a positive association between presleep cues (bedroom, routines, and habits) and a physiological and psychological state conducive to sleep. In addition, stimulus control recommendations aim to curtail counterproductive habits which may be used to try to cope with sleep disturbances such as sleeping in late or daytime napping in an effort to make up for lost sleep. Concerning daytime naps, although naps can be felt as necessary for many persons after TBI, even up to several years, it is important to consider the potential impact of naps on nighttime sleep. Naps during the day may diminish the sleep drive (which is linked to the length of the previous period of wakefulness). Taken too close to bedtime, a nap can delay sleep onset and make the nocturnal sleep lighter. Naps that are too long can produce sleep inertia, a feeling of grogginess that may have a negative impact on functioning for some time. Short naps (15–30 minutes) before 3:00 p.m. are thus recommended if the person feels the nap is necessary. In cases where the patient feels particularly sleep deprived, two separate short naps could be considered instead of one longer nap.

Stimulus control recommendations appear quite simple, however, the challenge for clinicians is to foster strict adherence with these instructions on the part of the patient. The clinician may need to help patients to implement these changes over several weeks, reiterating the importance of commitment and adherence to recommendations. To obtain more favorable outcomes, stimulus control instructions are ideally combined *with* the restriction of time in bed procedures. This can imply, for example, that a patient who does not feel sleepy at the bedtime suggested by the prescribed "sleep window" will wait until he or she feels some signs of sleepiness.

Implementation

Stimulus control therapy involves six key recommendations. The goal of these behavior changes is to regularize the sleep–wake rhythm and to reassociate temporal cues (bedtime) and environmental stimuli (bed and bedroom) with rapid sleep onset and well-being rather than cognitive, emotional, or physical tension related to sleep or to health-related worries. The recommendations are as follows:

- To reserve 1 hour before bedtime to create a relaxing presleep routine.
- To go to bed only when actually feeling sleepy (watching for objective signs of sleepiness such as yawning, eyelids drooping, dozing off—not merely feeling fatigued).
- To get out of bed when unable to sleep after about 20 minutes, ideally go to another room and return to bed only when feel sleepy again.
- To curtail sleep-incompatible activities such as watching television, using electronic devices, working, planning, worrying or problem-solving in the bed.
- To get up at a regular time every morning regardless of the amount of sleep and even on weekends.
- To avoid daytime napping.

Some TBI patients may encounter barriers to implementing these strategies; if, for example, they have pain or mobility issues and if leaving the bedroom is complex due to mobility issues or risks of fall, a comfortable chair or sofa can be used to slightly change the environment during nighttime awakenings (e.g., listen to music in a comfortable chair with a blanket while waiting for signs of sleepiness). For patients with marked post-TBI fatigue, naps are possibly difficult to avoid altogether. In these cases, however, some effort can be made to, for example, a short midafternoon nap (e.g., 15–30 minutes and starting no later than 3:00 p. m.). This flexible application of the recommendation may ease the process during the early phase of restriction of time in bed intervention or for patients who are markedly fatigued.

Brief Cognitive Therapy for Insomnia: Working on Unhelpful Thoughts, Beliefs, and Attitudes About Sleep and Insomnia

Rationale

Individuals suffering from insomnia may present several unhelpful thoughts, attitudes, or beliefs about sleep that contribute to maintain or even exacerbate their sleep disturbances. Examples include unrealistic expectations about sleep (e.g., "I absolutely need 8 hours of sleep to be functional during the day"), dysfunctional appraisals about sleep (I have completely lost control over my sleep), misattributions of daytime difficulties (e.g., blaming sleep or fatigue for everything that goes wrong during the day) (Morin, 1993), and misconceptions about the causes of insomnia (e.g., attributing insomnia exclusively to a physiological factor such as aging or pain). Patients recovering from TBI may entertain the same types of thoughts and beliefs (e.g., attributing insomnia exclusively to their brain injury), but in addition, they may be worried about the potential impact of sleep difficulties on their neural recuperation ("If I don't sleep well, my brain will not recover from my TBI"). The notion of rest can also be a source of pressure ("My caregivers tell me to rest and I can't do it. This is catastrophic," "If I cannot sleep well, I will never be able to return to work"). These types of thoughts can feed performance anxiety about sleep or can provoke negative emotions interfering with sleep onset. Such negative thoughts can be linked to negative emotions (fear, anxiety) that may contribute to somatic tension or cognitive arousal, which are incompatible with sleep, thus contributing to a vicious cycle. Negative thoughts might also arise during nighttime awakenings and may lead to monitoring behaviors such as clock watching to check how many hours are left in the night, or engaging with worries, which can prolong the nocturnal awakening.

Implementation

The original CBT for insomnia protocol proposed by Morin (1993) includes a cognitive therapy component aimed at modifying maladaptive thoughts, expectations, attitudes, beliefs, and cognitive processes (e.g., worrying, rumination) which contribute to the sleep disruption. This therapy component may be put into place with Socratic questioning and behavioral experiments. In the context of TBI, we have simplified this therapy component. One concrete way to implement this simplified version of cognitive therapy is to identify which unhelpful cognitions, beliefs, or attitudes the patient has endorsed on the dysfunctional beliefs and attitudes scale (DBAS, see Chapter 4: Assessment Tools for Post–TBI Insomnia) and to work from there. A first step might be to work with patients to identify the type of evidence (mostly personal experiences) supporting this belief and evidence not supporting it. If a traditional Socratic questioning approach is not feasible (e.g., with patients who have less insight or have difficulty with abstract reasoning), the following key messages (adapting the language as needed) can be conveyed to foster more realistic and helpful thought patterns.

- Although TBI and its symptoms may be responsible for having triggered insomnia, its maintenance over time is mainly due to behavioral and cognitive factors that the person can change. Even if some sleep-altering TBI symptoms persist and can cause nocturnal awakenings (e.g., pain), CBT for insomnia can still help in reducing the duration of these periods of wakefulness.
- It is important to keep realistic expectations with regard to sleep. In a context of insomnia, it is easy to think that all the impairments felt during the day, such as difficulty concentrating, sleepiness, or irritability, are due to poor sleep, but many factors may be at play.
- Never *try* to force sleep, this may exacerbate sleep difficulties with pressure and frustration.
- Do not give too much importance to sleep. Although sleep is an important part of a healthy life, it should not become the central point of attention.
- Avoid catastrophizing after a poor night. Although insomnia is quite unpleasant, it will not lead to direct effects on health at least not in the short term.
- Develop some tolerance to the effects of insomnia and prepare for setbacks. Everyone experiences occasional poor nights of sleep. Persons who are predisposed to insomnia remain more vulnerable to sleep disturbances even after a successful therapy. Occasional nights with insomnia are to be expected, but the strategies learned in therapy will help cope with these.

Presenting these arguments in written format is useful (see tools in Chapter 6), and it may help to verify the comprehension and retention of the information by patients and to repeat if necessary. The DBAS can also be filled out at several time points during the intervention to verify the evolution of beliefs and attitudes. If more elaborate cognitive therapy techniques for insomnia are feasible (e.g., identification of automatic thoughts, the Socratic questioning, downward arrow technique, and cost–benefit analysis), the clinician may refer to manuals developed for insomnia in the general population (Harvey, 2002, 2005; Morin, 1993; Morin & Espie, 2003) or to works on cognitive therapy per se (Beck, 2011; Bennett-Levy et al., 2004).

COGNITIVE–BEHAVIORAL THERAPY COMPONENTS SPECIFIC TO POST–TBI FATIGUE

Psychoeducation About Fatigue After Traumatic Brain Injury, and Health Habits Influencing Energy Levels

Rationale

Individuals with TBI often feel they were unprepared for the intensity and duration of fatigue which comes in the aftermath of the injury (Theadom et al., 2016). Because it is quite common and unfortunately often chronic (although the intensity and impacts can diminish over time), providing information about post-TBI fatigue may help to normalize the person's experience and predispose them to gradual adaptation to this newly acquired condition. When addressing fatigue, understanding how energy levels are linked to mood, physical activity, and other types of activities (e.g., social, housework) may encourage a more balanced planning of activities.

Implementation

While it is important for clinicians to normalize the experience of fatigue and to gently prepare patients for its potential chronic course, it is important to foster hope that the fatigue will decrease to a certain point and that the patient can learn to adapt and function satisfactorily despite its presence. It may help, for example, to explain that both physical and mental fatigue can occur, and even coexist, or fatigue may sometimes present as a general sensation of weariness. As such, even tasks that do not seem physically demanding, but that require planning or concentration, for example, may lead to fatigue, a phenomenon sometimes coined as *cognitive fatigability*. Gradually, the person will learn which activities are most demanding and need to be adapted or timed more appropriately. It is also important to distinguish fatigue (a subjective sense of lack of energy interfering with activities) from sleepiness (a physiological drive to sleep accompanied by signs such as eyelids drooping, yawning) which may also be present following TBI. Indeed, while sleepiness is a state conducive to sleep, fatigue is not necessarily. One might feel quite fatigued or tired without being able to fall asleep. Explaining the different factors that can influence energy levels (diet, exercise, mood, illness, etc.) can also help the patient decatastrophize the impacts of fatigue and envisage different potential ways to gain some control over this seemingly overwhelming symptom. Chapter 7 presents figures of a vicious cycle of fatigue followed by a positive cycle of energy management, as well as a list of lifestyle habits known to influence energy levels (e.g., diet, exercise, and stress). These tools may help normalize the person's experience, enhance comprehension of their problem, and support the perception that several factors and habits may be perpetuating fatigue over the long term, but that several of these can be modified in order to improve energy level.

Increasing Self-Awareness of Energy Levels and Signs of Fatigue

Rationale

Patients with TBI will often report that they sometimes will engage in a demanding activity for a given period of time, but then rather suddenly will feel exhausted and then may need to rest for an extended period of time (e.g., staying in bed a whole afternoon or even more) (Theadom et al., 2016). This may lead to cycles of overexertion followed by a significant need for rest, and eventually to avoid activities as a whole (which can lead to overall low levels of activity). Some clinicians and patients also refer to this phenomenon as the "Boom and Bust cycle" (Antcliff, Keeley, Campbell, Woby, & McGowan, 2016). In the TBI population, we hypothesize that these cycles suggest at least two things: (1) that the patient has not yet developed awareness of which types of activities are particularly demanding or will more readily lead to exhaustion (e.g., tasks combining a need for concentration and planning) and (2) that during any given activity, the patient may not consciously monitor his or her level of energy so as to manage his or her "energy bank" and as such does not consciously pace the activity as to avoid overdoing it.

Implementation

Although developing such an awareness of fatigue and learning how to pace activities may take time, rehabilitation professionals can help this process through simple exercises (Cantin et al., 2014). First, the patient is invited to identify what are his or her own signs of fatigue: these may include physical signs such as headaches or weariness, cognitive signs such as making mistakes, emotional signs such as irritability, and many others. The signs of one's fatigue may be explored first spontaneously, and if needed with the help of a checklist, ideally "live" during a given activity. For example, the patient can plan an activity known to be demanding and consciously monitor energy levels during the entire activity. The patient can also discuss signs of fatigue with a significant other. Indeed, it is not unusual for significant others to report that they need to cue the patient when they observe that he or she is overdoing an activity and needs to rest (Theadom et al., 2016).

Although such feedback from a significant other may help the patient better gauge energy levels in several instances, caution is warranted because this could also cause frictions (e.g., a spouse telling a patient that he or she is tired because he or she made an aggressive comment). As such, significant others may be invited to let patients develop their *self*-awareness, for example, by experiencing to a reasonable point of different levels of fatigue and by observing and discussing at an appropriate time the links between activities and energy levels.

Beyond the signs of fatigue, patients can be invited to list the different types of activities that compose their days and evaluate which activities are more or less demanding. This exercise might allow an individual to notice, for example, that tasks requiring sustained attention, sequencing, or planning (e.g., planning and preparing a meal, completing important paperwork) may be more demanding than others which are perhaps more automatic or require different types of energy (e.g., walking, washing dishes).

Activity Management or "Pacing" for Fatigue

Rationale

Early models of CBT for chronic fatigue syndrome underscored that fatigue led to a vicious cycle of inactivity in response to fatigue, with depression and physical deconditioning linked to inactivity feeding into the fatigue. Increasing physical activity levels was thus identified as the primary behavioral strategy to reduce fatigue (Wessely, David, Butler, & Chalder, 1989). Further work identified that beyond physical inactivity, persons with chronic fatigue also entertained negative thoughts and beliefs about engaging in a variety of activities (e.g., anticipating negative consequences) and developed recurrent thoughts about the need to rest (Surawy, Hackmann, Hawton, & Sharpe, 1995). In turn, these cognitive elements were thought to feed the person's inactivity in general: the person might limit their social, productive, leisure, and other types of activities. In parallel to the avoidance of some activities, individuals with chronic fatigue also naturally feel the need to meet their obligations and responsibilities. This may lead to bursts in activity when they feel well, and ensuing overexertion, thus exacerbating fatigue and causing a period of prolonged inactivity to recuperate.

The rationale of activity management or pacing is to gradually increase patients' level of activity, while taking into account the patient's capacities, to eventually arrive at a level that is more satisfactory for the patient. More precisely, activity management or pacing for fatigue aims at educating patient toward better energy management, with the aim of maximizing activities (these may be cognitive and/or physical) while avoiding overexertion (NICE, 2007). To achieve this, a person must be able to perceive one's own signs of exertion and to take a flexible approach to plan activities in order to stay with one's limits in terms of energy available. For persons who have sustained TBI (as in several other medical conditions, for example stroke), the fatigue may have developed quite abruptly. The process of learning to perceive the signs of fatigue is an important prerequisite step.

Implementation

Activity management or pacing is done by educating the patient about how activities can be adapted to accommodate fatigue. The idea is to be able to be active, despite the presence of fatigue, all the while respecting one's own limits and avoiding overexertion. Activity adaptation is done by planning activities realistically with the use of the following strategies:

- Planning rest periods in advance and identifying in advance *how* the person will rest (e.g., take a walk outside, listen to music);
- Dividing activities into shorter periods of time or more manageable units so as not to exacerbate fatigue; and
- Alternating between different types of tasks, one more demanding, another less demanding or of a different nature (e.g., alternate between a demanding cognitive task and a gentle physical task requiring little concentration).

The clinician may want to guide the patient in the planning of several activities in the upcoming week and to model how to self-monitor before, during, or after the activity. For example, more demanding or important tasks could be planned at the time of day when the person feels more energetic (in general in the morning for many patients) (Ouellet & Morin, 2006), while planning several breaks or manageable steps dispersed over several days. Once this planning is done, the patient is invited to follow through with several behavioral experiments where he or she will try to engage in these "adapted" activities, evaluate levels of energy during and after the activities (usually with the help of an energy/activity diary or a daily planner), notice thoughts and feelings during the activities, and globally note how these experiments went. Several weeks of experimentation with activity planning/evaluation may be necessary before the individual develops an adequate understanding of how energy fluctuates and how activities can be adapted to optimize energy levels.

Working on Attitudes About Fatigue

Rationale

Research examining the mediators of CBT for fatigue in multiple sclerosis and those of graded physical exercise in chronic fatigue syndrome (Knoop, van Kessel, & Moss-Morris, 2012; Wiborg, Knoop, Stulemeijer, Prins, & Bleijenberg, 2010) indicates that changes in *perceptions* of fatigue are a key therapeutic ingredient. Indeed, during therapy, the patient develops the perception that fatigue is more controllable, is a phenomenon that can be understood, and that it fluctuates with time. This change in the negative representation of fatigue has been shown to be even more predictive of treatment gains than behavioral changes such as increased physical activity or fitness. This underscores the need to specifically address patients' beliefs about fatigue and catastrophization.

Implementation

Post-TBI fatigue can seem overwhelming, and patients may feel they have no control over it. By first exploring the various factors influencing energy levels and fatigue, this may help the patient identify factors that are more seemingly controllable (e.g., sleep schedule, eating habits, medication use, and exercise). Through self-monitoring of activities, patients should be encouraged to notice what they are able to do in spite of fatigue, rather than focusing solely on what they are unable to do. They can also be invited to ponder on their own strategies to rest, and to broaden their definition of rest, by imagining different ways to rest even by being somewhat active (e.g., taking a short walk outside in sunlight, having a laugh with a friend, and listening to music). It is also useful for the patient to reflect upon the balance between different types of activities (e.g., obligations or responsibilities, social, physical, mental, pleasurable, and leisure activities) considering his or her valued roles and goals. This may help the person to reconsider how certain activities are prioritized and help to strive for a better balance between activities in order to contribute to self-esteem (e.g., productive tasks), social support and connectedness, and more globally mental and physical health. Throughout the intervention, and especially during activity management and pacing, the patient should be encouraged to maintain realistic expectations about energy levels and can reflect upon situations where it is acceptable to ask for help, delegate, shorten, or adapt the activity. Chapter 7 includes tools to support these strategies. As the situation and activities of the patient may change (e.g., gradual return to work), these tools could be completed several times at different stages in the patient's community reintegration trajectory. Finally, patients might have completely stopped certain activities they appreciated before the injury because of fatigue. Despite potential newly acquired limitations (e.g., motor limitations, cognitive issues), if the patient seems ready for this, the clinician may want to invite the patient to explore how to reintegrate avoided activities with potential adaptations (which can be as simple as trying the activity for 15 minutes), the goal being for the person to become aware that they might find pleasure or gratification in these activities even if adapted. The clinician may invite the patient to put aside any comparison with before the injury and to consider the activity as a new version (2.0 version) to foster openness to the adapted experience. If such previously appreciated activities are no longer possible in any way, exploring and integrating new activities (e.g., new leisure, social, or exercise activities) can be another option, again considering the patient's values and goals (referral to an occupational therapist or leisure specialist may should be considered). These shifts in attitudes may give way to a gradual increase in activity levels for patients.

ADDITIONAL COMPONENTS

Encouraging Graded Physical Exercise

Rationale

Exercise has beneficial effects on sleep quality, quantity, and in reducing fatigue in a variety of populations (Hilfiker et al., 2018; Kelley & Kelley, 2017), although the evidence for TBI per se is still quite limited (Xu, Li, Wang, & Cao, 2017). For example, a recent Cochrane systematic review (Larun, Brurberg, Odgaard-Jensen, & Price, 2017) indicates that patients with chronic fatigue syndrome feel significantly less fatigued following exercise therapy, and furthermore seem to improve on measures of sleep, physical functioning, and general health. Even a simple, accessible and free activity such as walking (in the absence of gait impairments) can have measurable benefits (Kolakowsky-Hayner et al., 2017).

Implementation

Having evaluated the patient's current exercise habits and verified any potential contraindications or recommendations issued by other health professionals (e.g., orthopedic condition limiting potential activities), the goal is to gradually augment the duration and/or intensity of exercise starting from the patient's baseline level of activity. For example, a simple specific and achievable goal can be agreed upon with the patient for exercise during the following week. The patient should be able to complete their goal even on a "bad day." The clinician may consider referral to an exercise professional as needed and recommendations should not be made without a medical confirmation that the type of physical activity is appropriate for the patient.

Stress and Worry Management

Rationale

Although providing stress-management tools goes beyond the scope of this manual, it is important not to dismiss the important role of worrying, rumination, and somatic tension in sleep difficulties and fatigue after TBI. Indeed, increased physiological, cognitive, or emotional activation can cause fatigue during the day as well as difficulties to fall asleep (Morin, 1993). For example, worries about certain subjects such as overall health, recovery, and capacity to work, finances or litigation may have become overwhelming for patients.

Implementation

One strategy to minimize rumination or worrying at bedtime is to suggest patients set aside a specific time and place (other than bedtime and the bedroom) where they allow themselves to worry, problem-solving, plan, or simply write down more negative thoughts or emotions. Ideally, this period should be planned in advance and clearly defined with a beginning and ending time. The patient is encouraged to postpone to his "worry time/place" major concerns or worries that come to mind at other times during the day. These can be noted down while reminding oneself that this concern will be dealt with later, and more efficiently, during the worry period. The patient can also remind him or herself that attending to the present tasks will lead to more satisfaction and/or well-being. Patients can also be instructed with specific relaxation, mindfulness, or imagery techniques to manage activating presleep thoughts or worries during the day.

Involving a Family Member

Rationale

Collaboration between the clinician and the patient's family/friends is essential. Certain attitudes from significant others may undermine clinician and patient efforts during and after intervention for insomnia or fatigue. Following are a few examples:

- Encouraging the patient to go to bed earlier than his or her sleep window because the patient feels tired or irritable;

- Encouraging the patient to take naps at any time of day because he or she feels tired or irritable;
- Canceling appointments or social occasions to let the patient rest;
- Constantly taking care of tasks that are too tiring for the patient, instead of allowing him or her to learn to perform these tasks through better energy management (e.g., breaking down tasks into steps, prioritizing tasks, or alternating between different types of tasks). In this case the family member or friend may also become exhausted;
- Systematically attributing problems such as patient irritability, difficulties with concentration or memory, organization problems, or aggressiveness to a lack of sleep or to post-TBI fatigue;
- Perceiving the patient's fatigue as laziness or a lack of willpower;
- Refusing to change one's own habits in connection with the sleep−wake cycle (e.g., watching TV in bed, insisting in going to bed too early) when these habits appear to be contributing the patient's sleep or fatigue problem;
- Discouraging the patient from engaging in physical exercise out of a fear that he or she will fall down and sustain another injury;
- Encouraging the patient to use frequent medication or substances (e.g., alcohol or marijuana) as a sleep aid or to help him or her be more awake or active during the day (e.g., energy drinks, coffee, soft drinks containing caffeine);
- Contributing to an environment conducive to wakefulness (e.g., noise, snoring, moving around, and higher temperatures); and
- Systematically eating meals that are too heavy, soon before bedtime, or accompanied by too much alcohol.

Implementation

Ask the patient if he or she can enlist the support of family/friends (e.g., a spouse, a friend, a parent, or a child). For patients with severe cognitive impairments or behavioral challenges, it can be useful to invite one or more family members or friends to attend certain appointments. In this way the family member or friend will become aware of the impact of the patient's sleep difficulties, the rationale behind certain interventions and recommendations, and the importance of applying recommendations diligently. Indeed, the intervention can lead to changes in habits or lifestyles which also concern a spouse or other members of the household. If everyone involved understands the rationale of the intervention, the client will likely receive more support and encouragement during the therapeutic process. Major role changes may have occurred postinjury: for example, a spouse can have taken over a large number of household chores after the accident for fear of "fatiguing" their loved one with TBI. This behavior, although well-intentioned and useful up to a certain limit, can undermine the efforts made to reactivate the client if very fatigued. Similarly, significant others may cancel the patient's medical, social, or work-related appointments because their loved one is too tired or has had a poor night of sleep. For a spouse who likes to read or listen to the television in bed before turning off the lights, eliminating such a habit can be difficult for those who do not have trouble sleeping. However, if the deleterious effects of this practice are explained to him or her while seeking his support, he or she will probably be more cooperative and encouraging.

CLINICAL CHALLENGES IN THE CONTEXT OF TRAUMATIC BRAIN INJURY

As with most physical and psychological health conditions, a number of factors need to be considered when assessing or beginning psychological treatment for insomnia or fatigue with people who have suffered from TBI. Following are some of the factors to keep in mind in order to adapt elements of this manual to the TBI context.

Cognitive Impairment

Due to cognitive impairment (memory, attention, or communication problems), some clients with TBI might have difficulty grasping the rationale of certain recommendations or have problems encoding and retaining information presented in therapy. The following strategies can be used to minimize the effects of cognitive impairment:

- As needed, take more time to explain the rationale for a recommendation and illustrate with examples.
- Make sure that the patient understands the rationale of a treatment recommendation by asking him or her to explain it in his or her words. This will enhance the encoding and retention of the information, as well as adherence to treatment strategies.
- Adapt language as needed: use concrete examples, illustrations, pictures, diagrams, or metaphors (e.g., presenting one's energy banks as a battery, a bank account, or a traffic light).
- Repeat information over multiple sessions.
- Ask the client to explain the rationale for a recommendation to one of their relatives.
- Present information both verbally and visually (print the tools).

- Suggest shorter appointments, or vary their duration depending on the complexity of the material presented.
- Provide simplified texts, diagrams, or illustrations.
- Model self-monitoring: fill out and interpret suggested tools together with patients (e.g., sleep diary).
- Shorten or adapt suggested tools.
- Consider in-between telephone calls or emails to remind the client of prescribed recommendations or homework.
- End sessions with a summary and ask clients to record the key points to remember and to apply until the next session (e.g., using a notebook or mobile device).
- Get a third party involved in helping and supporting the patient during the assessment and intervention process (e.g., his or her partner). In this case, however, it is important to familiarize this other individual with the rationale behind interventions.

Behavioral Particularities

Following through with these treatments can be more challenging when working with patients exhibiting behavioral problems. Indeed, some patients may have difficulties with planning and organization (this can, for example, lead to more missed appointments), others may present with impulsiveness or lack of initiative, or use of consumption of recreational drugs and alcohol. The following strategies can be used to minimize the impact of behavioral particularities on the effectiveness of the intervention:

- Take into account the education and literacy level of patients and adapt intervention as needed.
- Discuss the importance of filling out assessment tools or applying therapeutic recommendations while maintaining flexibility.
- Provide proper guidance that takes into account the variety of services already received.
- Explain interactions between substance use and problems with sleep and fatigue. Monitor substance use throughout treatment (e.g., using a sleep/energy diary). Consider referring patients with significant problems with substance use, or discontinuing treatment if it is drastically impeded.
- Explore what the patient is willing to do (for example with motivational interviewing techniques).
- Encourage the use of reminders and other tools for planning (e.g., smartphone, paper, or electronic calendar).

Physical Impairment

Pain, mobility limitations, and physical deconditioning may interfere with the implementation of CBT interventions for insomnia and fatigue. The following strategies can be helpful:

- Stay in touch with physicians and other health professionals in order to assess the potential role of pain, mobility limitations, and physical functioning in the patient's insomnia or fatigue, and to explore the patient's range of potential activities.
- Make sure that pain is properly controlled and keep a note of any medication prescribed to the patient for pain or other problems. For instance, opioids prescribed for pain can cause daytime sleepiness and interfere with compliance (e.g., excessive napping, inactivity, using the bed or bedroom for daytime sleep or rest).
- Discuss with the patient about his or her perceptions and beliefs regarding the interaction between pain, physical functioning, sleep, and fatigue.
- Include interventions aimed at modifying pain and physical limitation management strategies when these strategies interfere with sleep or energy levels.

Polypharmacy and Sleep Medication

It is useful to be familiar with the potential effects of medication taken by the patient for sleep, fatigue, pain, cognition, psychological symptoms, and neurological conditions (e.g., epilepsy). Some medications can lead to or exacerbate sleep or fatigue problems. It is essential to be in communication with the attending physician if a prescribed medication or drug interaction appears to be adversely affecting sleep or provoking issues with daytime sleepiness or fatigue.

Many individuals with sleep difficulties take prescribed or over-the-counter medications to manage their sleep. Using medication is not a contraindication for applying the CBT intervention components suggested in this manual. To the contrary, behavioral recommendations can be applied while continuing to use medication. It is often useful for patients to start by applying the behavioral strategies, and experience their beneficial effects, before ceasing their medication. This strategy also allows the patient to focus on one change at a time and helps clarifying the attributions of therapeutic gains. If the patient wishes to stop using a medication, it is absolutely essential to make sure that tapering is gradual, follows a well-planned schedule, and takes place over several weeks, under the supervision of a doctor or pharmacist. These precautions are necessary in order to limit symptoms of tapering and to avoid exacerbating the insomnia.

Symptoms of Anxiety and Depression

Patients showing symptoms of depression and anxiety should be assessed carefully. Although studies tend to demonstrate that treating sleep and fatigue can have positive impacts on anxiety and mood (Belleville, Cousineau, Levrier, & St-Pierre-Delorme, 2011), caution is necessary:

- Address anxiety- and depression-related issues with the patient. It is very important to direct the patient to appropriate resources if the severity of psychiatric symptoms necessitates urgent treatment or when anxiety and depression appear to be the main clinical manifestation.
- Avoid undertaking insomnia intervention that includes limiting time spent in bed in the event of an acute and unstable psychological condition.
- Explain the connection between sleep, fatigue, depression, anxiety, and other related factors (e.g., pain).
- Encourage a balance between activities (physical, rewarding, useful, social, restful, pleasant activities, and rest).
- Encourage patients to regularly schedule pleasurable and/or satisfying activities to foster a sense of mastery and positive reinforcement regularly.
- Encourage the patient to use and expand his or her social support network.

Issues With Adherence and Motivation

Patients with TBI may have issues with organization, planning, initiative, and behavioral regulation. As such, it can be very difficult for patients to strictly apply certain recommendations proposed for sleep or fatigue. A flexible approach might be necessary, for example, by simplifying the recommendation at first, especially in the early stages, while keeping the goal or underlying rationale in mind. For example, if restriction of time in bed is difficult to implement, the recommendation could be simplified to explaining to the patient and significant other to try going to bed later and to arise in the morning at a regular time to avoid spending too much time awake in bed.

Some patients may also be reluctant to incorporate recommendations into their lifestyle. In these cases, consider applying a motivational approach, asking the patient what he or she would be willing to change. Another strategy is to collaboratively develop a hierarchy of behavioral changes, starting with the easiest change to incorporate into the patient's lifestyle, eventually aiming to fully implement the recommendations. Providing more encouragement or structure for patients who have issues with adherence is useful, as is reminding them that results are often not noticed until the recommendations have been incorporated for a certain period of time.

References

Antcliff, D., Keeley, P., Campbell, M., Woby, S., & McGowan, L. (2016). Exploring patients' opinions of activity pacing and a new activity pacing questionnaire for chronic pain and/or fatigue: A qualitative study. *Physiotherapy, 102*(3), 300–307. Available from https://doi.org/10.1016/j.physio.2015.08.001.

Beck, J. S. (2011). *Cognitive therapy: Basics and beyond* (2nd ed.). New York: Guilford Press.

Belleville, G., Cousineau, H., Levrier, K., & St-Pierre-Delorme, M. E. (2011). Meta-analytic review of the impact of cognitive-behavior therapy for insomnia on concomitant anxiety. *Clinical Psychology Review, 31*(4), 638–652. Available from https://doi.org/10.1016/j.cpr.2011.02.004.

Bennett-Levy, J., Butler, G., Fennell, M., Hackman, A., Mueller, M., & Westbrook, D. (2004). *Cognitive behaviour therapy: Science and practice series. Oxford guide to behavioural experiments in cognitive therapy.* New York: Oxford University Press.

Cantin, J.-F., Ouellet, M.-C., Turcotte, N., Lessard, J., Potvin, I., Boutin, N., & Duchesneau, G. (2014). *Le guide de l'énergie: vers une meilleure gestion de la fatigue.* Québec: Institut de réadaptation en déficience physique de Québec.

Cohen, J. S., Edmunds, J. M., Brodman, D. M., Benjamin, C. L., & Kendall, P. C. (2013). Using self-monitoring: Implementation of collaborative empiricism in cognitive-behavioral therapy. *Cognitive and Behavioral Practice, 20*(4), 419–428.

Harvey, A. G. (2002). A cognitive model of insomnia. *Behaviour Research and Therapy, 40*(8), 869–893. Retrieved from <http://www.ncbi.nlm.nih.gov/pubmed/12186352>.

Harvey, A. G. (2005). A cognitive theory and therapy for chronic insomnia. *Journal of Cognitive Psychotherapy, 19*, 41–59.

Hilfiker, R., Meichtry, A., Eicher, M., Nilsson Balfe, L., Knols, R. H., Verra, M. L., & Taeymans, J. (2018). Exercise and other non-pharmaceutical interventions for cancer-related fatigue in patients during or after cancer treatment: A systematic review incorporating an indirect-comparisons meta-analysis. *British Journal of Sports Medicine, 52* (10), 651–658. Available from https://doi.org/10.1136/bjsports-2016-096422.

Kelley, G. A., & Kelley, K. S. (2017). Exercise and sleep: A systematic review of previous meta-analyses. *Journal of Evidence-Based Medicine, 10*(1), 26–36. Available from https://doi.org/10.1111/jebm.12236.

Knoop, H., van Kessel, K., & Moss-Morris, R. (2012). Which cognitions and behaviours mediate the positive effect of cognitive behavioural therapy on fatigue in patients with multiple sclerosis? *Psychological Medicine, 42*(1), 205–213. Available from https://doi.org/10.1017/s0033291711000924.

Kolakowsky-Hayner, S. A., Bellon, K., Toda, K., Bushnik, T., Wright, J., Isaac, L., & Englander, J. (2017). A randomised control trial of walking to ameliorate brain injury fatigue: A NIDRR TBI model system centre-based study. *Neuropsychological Rehabilitation, 27*(7), 1002–1018. Available from https://doi.org/10.1080/09602011.2016.1229680.

Larun, L., Brurberg, K. G., Odgaard-Jensen, J., & Price, J. R. (2017). Exercise therapy for chronic fatigue syndrome. *Cochrane Database of Systematic Reviews, 4*, Cd003200. Available from https://doi.org/10.1002/14651858.CD003200.pub7.

Miller, C. B., Espie, C. A., Epstein, D. R., Friedman, L., Morin, C. M., Pigeon, W. R., ... Kyle, S. D. (2014). The evidence base of sleep restriction therapy for treating insomnia disorder. *Sleep Medicine Reviews*, *18*(5), 415–424. Available from https://doi.org/10.1016/j.smrv.2014.01.006.

Morgenthaler, T., Kramer, M., Alessi, C., Friedman, L., Boehlecke, B., Brown, T., ... Lichstein, K. L. (2006). Practice parameters for the psychological and behavioral treatment of insomnia: An update. An American Academy of Sleep Medicine report.

Morin, C. (1993). *Insomnia: Psychological assessment and management*. New York: Guilford.

Morin, C. M., & Espie, C. A. (2003). *Insomnia: A clinical guide to assessment and treatment*. New York: Kluwer Academic/Plenum.

NICE. *Chronic fatigue syndrome/myalgic encephalomyelitis (or encephalopathy): Diagnosis and management (Clinical Guideline CG53)*. (2007). Retrieved from <https://www.nice.org.uk/guidance/cg53>.

Ouellet, M.-C., & Morin, C. M. (2006). Fatigue following traumatic brain injury: Frequency, characteristics, and associated factors. *Rehabilitation Psychology*, *51*, 140–149. Available from https://doi.org/10.1037/0090-5550.51.2.140.

Spielman, A. J., Saskin, P., & Thorpy, M. J. (1987). Treatment of chronic insomnia by restriction of time in bed. *Sleep*, *10*(1), 45–56. Retrieved from <http://www.ncbi.nlm.nih.gov/entrez/query.fcgi?cmd = Retrieve&db = PubMed&dopt = Citation&list_uids = 3563247>.

Surawy, C., Hackmann, A., Hawton, K., & Sharpe, M. (1995). Chronic fatigue syndrome: A cognitive approach. *Behaviour Research and Therapy*, *33*(5), 535–544.

Theadom, A., Rowland, V., Levack, W., Starkey, N., Wilkinson-Meyers, L., & McPherson, K. (2016). Exploring the experience of sleep and fatigue in male and female adults over the 2 years following traumatic brain injury: A qualitative descriptive study. *BMJ Open*, *6*(4), e010453. Available from https://doi.org/10.1136/bmjopen-2015-010453.

Wessely, S., David, A., Butler, S., & Chalder, T. (1989). Management of chronic (post-viral) fatigue syndrome. *The Journal of the Royal College of General Practitioners*, *39*(318), 26–29.

Wiborg, J. F., Knoop, H., Stulemeijer, M., Prins, J. B., & Bleijenberg, G. (2010). How does cognitive behaviour therapy reduce fatigue in patients with chronic fatigue syndrome? The role of physical activity. *Psychological Medicine*, *40*(8), 1281–1287. Available from https://doi.org/10.1017/s0033291709992212.

Xu, G. Z., Li, Y. F., Wang, M. D., & Cao, D. Y. (2017). Complementary and alternative interventions for fatigue management after traumatic brain injury: A systematic review. *Therapeutic Advances in Neurological Disorders*, *10*(5), 229–239. Available from https://doi.org/10.1177/1756285616682675.

PRACTICAL TOOLS

Assessment Tools for Post-TBI Insomnia

OVERVIEW

This chapter is a compendium of assessment tools for post-TBI insomnia. It includes the following tools and clinician guides:

- DSM-5 Diagnostic criteria for an insomnia disorder
- Clinical Interview on Insomnia following traumatic brain injury (full version)
- Clinical Interview on Insomnia following traumatic brain injury (short version)
- Sleep diary (full version)
- Sleep diary—Example and instructions
- Sleep diary—Short version
- Sleep diary—Analysis
- Sleep diary—How to compute sleep efficiency
- Insomnia Severity Index (ISI)
- Insomnia Severity Index (ISI)—Scoring and interpretation
- Dysfunctional Beliefs and Attitudes About Sleep (DBAS)
- Dysfunctional Beliefs and Attitudes About Sleep (DBAS)—Scoring and interpretation
- Case Conceptualization summary for post-TBI Insomnia

Clinician guide
DSM-5 Diagnostic Criteria for an Insomnia Disorder

A. A predominant complaint of dissatisfaction with sleep quantity or quality, associated with one (or more) of the following symptoms: 1. Difficulty initiating sleep. 2. Difficulty maintaining sleep, characterized by frequent awakenings or problems returning to sleep after awakenings. 3. Early morning awakening with inability to return to sleep.
B. The sleep disturbance causes clinically significant distress or impairment in social, occupational, educational, academic, behavioral, or other important areas of functioning.
C. The sleep difficulty occurs at least 3 nights per week.
D. The sleep difficulty is present for at least 3 months.
E. The sleep difficulty occurs despite adequate opportunity for sleep.
F. The insomnia is not better explained by and does not occur exclusively during the course of another sleep–wake disorder (e.g., narcolepsy, a breathing-related sleep disorder, a circadian rhythm sleep–wake disorder, a parasomnia).
G. The insomnia is not attributable to the physiological effects of a substance (e.g., a drug of abuse, a medication).
H. Coexisting mental disorders and medical conditions do not adequately explain the predominant complaint of insomnia.
Specify if With nonsleep disorder mental comorbidity, including substance use disorders With other medical comorbidity With other sleep disorder
Specify if Episodic: Symptoms last at least 1 month but less than 3 months. Persistent: Symptoms last 3 months or longer. Recurrent: Two (or more) episodes in the space of 1 year.

Source: *From American Psychiatric Association. (2013). Diagnostic and statistical manual of mental disorders (5th ed.). Washington, DC: Author. Reprinted with permission from the Diagnostic and Statistical Manual of Mental Disorders, Fifth Edition, (Copyright 2013). American Psychiatric Association. All Rights Reserved.*

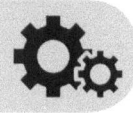

Clinical Interview on Insomnia Following Traumatic Brain Injury—Full Version

ID:	Date:

I. HISTORY OF SLEEP DIFFICULTIES:

1. For how long have you been having sleep difficulties?

_____

2. Did you have sleep difficulties before suffering a TBI?   ☐ Yes   ☐ No

3. Did your sleep change following the TBI?   ☐ Yes   ☐ No

    If so, describe the changes you have observed:

    During the acute phase/hospitalization:

    _____

    The first few weeks/months at home:

    _____

    When returning to your preinjury activities (family roles, work, studies, leisure, etc.):

    _____

4. Are there any stressful events which you associate with the onset of your sleep difficulties? (past or present difficulties)

    _____
    _____

5. Did your sleep difficulties begin suddenly or gradually?

    _____
    _____

6. How have your sleep difficulties evolved since they have started (persistent, episodic, seasonal)?

_____

_____

7. What do you think is the cause of your current sleep difficulties (e.g., worries, stress, pain, depression, medication, noise, environmental factors, schedule, or nothing in particular)?

_____

_____

8. In the past, have you ever received medications or other forms of therapy for sleep difficulties? Did these treatments prove useful?

   If so, specify type/duration/results:

_____

_____

II. SEVERITY OF INSOMNIA:

For this series of questions, refer to the past month.

9. What is your usual bedtime?   _____

10. What time is your last awakening in the morning   _____
    (without going back to sleep)?

11. What time do you usually get out of bed?   _____

12. Is your sleep schedule generally stable?   ☐ Yes   ☐ No
    (e.g., weekends, rotating shifts)?

    If not, how does it vary?   _____

13. Do you have difficulty falling asleep?   ☐ Yes   ☐ No

14. How long does it take you to fall asleep?   _____

15. In the past month, how many nights per week, on   _____ nights/week
    average, did you need more than 30 minutes to fall
    asleep?

16. Do you have difficulty staying asleep at night?   ☐ Yes   ☐ No

17. How many times per night do you wake up?   _____times/night

18. How much time, on average, do you spend awake   _____
    per night? (add up the duration of all awakenings)

19. How many nights per week, on average, do you   _____nights/week
    awake for more than 30 minutes in total?

20. What wakes you up at night?   _____
    (e.g., pain, noise, no specific reason)

21. Do you wake up too early in the morning?   ☐ Yes   ☐ No

22. How long before your desired time do you generally _____
    wake up in the morning? (e.g., before your alarm
    clock goes off)

23. How many nights per week, on average, do you wake up more than 30 minutes before your desired time?　　_____nights/week

24. Do you feel your sleep is not restorative?　　☐ Yes　　☐ No

25. How many nights per week, on average, do you feel that your sleep is not restorative?　　_____

26. How many hours do you sleep per night?　　_____hours/night

27. In the past month, how satisfied have you been with the quality of your sleep?　　_____

28. In the past month, how concerned have you been about your sleep difficulties?　　_____

III. DAYTIME FUNCTIONING:

For this series of questions, again please refer to the past month.

29. Do you have difficulty staying awake during the day? ☐ Yes ☐ No

30. Do you ever fall asleep at inappropriate times or in inappropriate places? If so, specify: ☐ Yes ☐ No

_____

31. In the past month, how many times per day did you fall asleep or doze off unintentionally? _____times/day

32. Do you take intentional naps during the day? ☐ Yes ☐ No

33. How many times per week do you take naps? _____times/week

34. What is the average duration of your naps? _____

35. Before your accident, would you take naps? _____

36. Do your sleep difficulties cause or worsen the following symptoms?

   a) Fatigue or low energy ☐ Yes ☐ No

   b) Difficulty with concentration, attention, or memory ☐ Yes ☐ No

   c) Reduced motivation or initiative ☐ Yes ☐ No

   d) Pain or headache ☐ Yes ☐ No

   e) Physical discomfort such as muscle tension or heartburn ☐ Yes ☐ No

   f) Sleepiness or difficulty staying awake or staying vigilant ☐ Yes ☐ No

   g) Irritability or impatience (anger, aggressiveness) ☐ Yes ☐ No

   h) Other effects?_____ ☐ Yes ☐ No

IV. ENVIRONMENT AND LIFESTYLE:

For this series of questions, again please refer to the past month.

37. Is your sleep environment comfortable?   ☐ Yes   ☐ No
    (e.g., bed, mattress, lighting, temperature, noise)

38. How many times per week do you exercise?   _____times/week

39. At what time(s) of the day do you typically exercise?   _____

40. How many caffeinated products do you consume   _____
    each day? *(e.g., coffee, energy drinks, carbonated drinks)*

41. How many cigarettes do you smoke per day?   _____

42. Do you smoke before bedtime?   ☐ Yes   ☐ No

43. Do you smoke during the night?   ☐ Yes   ☐ No

44. How many alcoholic drinks do you have in a typical   _____
    day or week since your injury?

45. Do you take recreational drugs?   ☐ Yes   ☐ No

    If so, specify:

    _____

46. How many times per day or week do you take   _____
    drugs?

47. In the past month, have you used   ☐ Yes   ☐ No
    alcohol or recreational drugs to help you sleep?
    Specify:_____

48. How many nights per week do you use alcohol or   _____nights/week
    recreational drugs to help you sleep?

V. HISTORY OF TREATMENTS FOR SLEEP DIFFICULTIES:

49. What strategies are you currently using to improve your sleep?

_____

_____

50. In the past month, have you used prescription or over-the-counter medication to help you sleep? ☐ Yes ☐ No

If so, specify (type, dose, etc.): _____

_____

51. How many nights per week do you take medication to sleep? _____nights/week

52. In the past, have you used prescription or over-the-counter medication to help you sleep? ☐ Yes ☐ No

If so, specify (type, dose, etc.): _____

_____

53. In the past month, have you used other types of treatments for sleep difficulties? ☐ Yes ☐ No

If so, specify: _____

_____

VI. SYMPTOMS ASSOCIATED WITH OTHER SLEEP DISORDERS:

54. Have you or your bed partner noticed any of the following symptoms?

	Specify the nature, frequency, and severity of symptoms, and contribution to sleep difficulties
Restless legs: Crawling or tingling sensation in your legs, urge to move your legs, and inability to keep legs still.	
Periodic limb movements: Jerking or twitching of your legs during the night, awakening with leg cramps.	
Apnea: Snoring, breathing difficulties, pauses in breathing, shortness of breath, chest pain, waking up with headaches or dry mouth.	
Narcolepsy: Sleep attacks (falling asleep suddenly and uncontrollably), sleep paralysis, hypnagogic hallucinations, cataplexy.	
Parasomnia: Nightmares, night terrors, bruxism (teeth grinding), walking or talking during sleep.	

VII. COMORBIDITY:

55. Do the following elements apply to your situation? If so, how much do they contribute to your sleep difficulties?
(In other words, would you have trouble sleeping even without these problems?)

	Specify the nature, frequency, and severity of issues	How do these contribute to your sleep difficulties?
Anxiety, nervousness, worrying		
Depression, sadness, loss of interest		
Alcohol or recreational drug use		
Pain		
Medical problem		
Prescription or over-the-counter medication (other than for sleep)		

 Clinical Interview on Insomnia Following Traumatic Brain Injury—Short Version

ID:	Date:

For the following series of questions, refer to the past month.

1. How long have you had sleep difficulties? (specify if these started before or after the TBI)
   Did your sleep change following the TBI?

   _____

2. Do you have difficulty falling asleep?   ☐ Yes,_____times/week   ☐ No

3. Do you have difficulty staying asleep at night?   ☐ Yes,_____times/week   ☐ No

4. Do you wake up too early in the morning?   ☐ Yes,_____times/week   ☐ No

5. How many hours do you sleep per night?   _____hours/night

6. Do you have difficulty staying awake during the day?   ☐ Yes   ☐ No

7. How many times per day or week do you fall asleep, intentionally or unintentionally?_____

8. How worried are you about your insomnia? *(on a scale of 1–10; 1 = not at all worried; 10 = extremely worried)*_____

   What do you worry about:

   _____

9. How does your insomnia affect your everyday life?

   _____

10. Does your insomnia affect people around you?

_____

11. Have you or your bed partner noticed any of the following symptoms? If so, how often do you experience them, and to what extent do they contribute to your sleep difficulties?
    (In other words, would you have difficulty sleeping even without these symptoms?)

    ☐ Loud snoring_____

    ☐ Pause in breathing while asleep_____

    ☐ Crawling sensations, with the urge to move your legs when going to bed_____

    ☐ Jerking or twitching of your legs during sleep_____

    ☐ Nightmares_____

    ☐ Other symptoms_____

    ☐ Pain_____

    ☐ Stress or anxiety_____

    ☐ Depressed mood_____

12. What strategies do you use to improve your sleep or your level of energy during the day? (e.g., prescription or over-the-counter medication, other substances, exercise, or other strategies)

_____

13. Is your sleep environment comfortable? (e.g., bed, mattress, lighting, temperature, noise)?

_____

Sleep Diary

- Fill out the sleep diary **every morning**.
- **Do not watch the clock** to fill out the diary: it is not important to get exact numbers, but rather your best **estimates**.

ID : _____

	Date	Date	Date	Date	Date	Date	Date
1. Yesterday, I napped from _____ to _____. (record the times for all naps)							
2. I got into bed at _____ (record the time)							
3. I tried to go to sleep at _____. (record the time)							
4. After turning the lights off, it took me _____ minutes to fall asleep.							
5. My sleep was interrupted _____ times. (record the number of awakenings)							
6. In total, my sleep was interrupted for _____ minutes. (record the total duration for all awakenings)							
7. Last night, I got out of bed _____ times. (record the number of times you got out of bed)							
8. This morning, my final awakening was at ___. (record the time of your final awakening without going back to sleep)							
9. This morning, I got out of bed at ___. (record the time)							
10. The quality of my sleep from last night was. (1–5; 1 = very bad; 5 = very good)							
11. Yesterday, I took _____ to help me sleep. (e.g., medication, alcohol, drug, natural product)							

Sleep Diary (Full Version)—Example and Instructions

ID : _____

		Date	
		July 9	
1.	Yesterday, I napped from _____ to _____. (record the times for all naps)	10–10:15 a.m. 3:30–4 p.m.	↵ Record the start time and end time of all naps, even if unintentional (e.g., falling asleep in front of the TV).
2.	I got into bed at _____. (record the time)	10:15 p.m.	↵ Record the time you went to bed.
3.	I tried to go to sleep at _____. (record the time)	10:30 p.m.	↵ Record the time when you tried to go to sleep (can be identical to or different from bedtime).
4.	After turning the lights off, it took me _____ minutes to fall asleep.	15 min	↵ Give your best estimate of the time you took to fall asleep after you began trying to do so.
5.	My sleep was interrupted _____ times. (record the number of awakenings)	2	↵ Estimate the number of times you woke up during the night.
6.	In total, my sleep was interrupted for _____ minutes. (record the total duration for all awakenings)	1 hr 30 min	↵ Estimate how much time you spent awake in total for all the times you woke up. Do not include your final awakening.
7.	Last night, I got out of bed _____ times. (record the number of times you got out of bed)	1	↵ Record the number of times you got out of bed during the night.
8.	This morning, my final awakening was at _____. (record the time of your final awakening without going back to sleep)	6:15 a.m.	↵ Record the final time you woke up without going back to sleep.
9.	This morning, I got out of bed at _____. (record the time)	7:00 a.m.	↵ Record the time you got out of bed for the day.
10.	The quality of my sleep from last night was _____. (1 to 5; 1 = very bad; 5 = very good)	3	↵ Estimate the overall quality of your sleep on a scale from 1–5.
11.	Yesterday, I took _____ to help me sleep. (e.g., medication, alcohol, drug, natural product)	Zopiclone 7.5 mg	↵ Record any medication or substances you used to help you fall sleep last night.

Sleep Diary—Short Version

- Fill out the sleep diary **every morning**.
- **Do not watch the clock** to fill out the diary: it is not important to get exact numbers, but rather your best **estimates**.

Date							
Bedtime							
Time taken to fall asleep							
Time spent awake during the night (total for all awakenings)							
Rising time							

Date							
Bedtime							
Time taken to fall asleep							
Time spent awake during the night (total for all awakenings)							
Rising time							

Clinician guide
Sleep Diary—Analysis

SLEEP SCHEDULE AND TIME SPENT IN BED	• Is the patient's sleep schedule (bedtime, rising time) stable or variable? (e.g., different on weekends) • Is the patient's sleep schedule adapted to his or her situation? • Does the patient spend a lot of time in bed before trying to fall asleep (time between bedtime and the time the patient tries to fall asleep) or after his or her final awakening?
TIME SPENT AWAKE DURING THE NIGHT	• Does the patient have difficulty falling asleep (time falling asleep >30 minutes, several times per week)? • Does the patient have difficulty staying asleep (total for all awakenings >30 minutes, several times per week)? • Does the patient wake up too early in the morning (time of final awakening >30 minutes before desired time, with insufficient total sleep time, several times per week)? • Is there significant night-to-night variability in the duration of awakenings?
TOTAL SLEEP TIME Time spent in bed minus total time awake	• Does the patient's total sleep time per night appear sufficient to meet his or her needs? • Is there significant night-to-night variability in total sleep time?
SLEEP EFFICIENCY Percentage of time in bed that the patient is asleep	• Overall, does the patient spend much more time in bed compared to the total sleep time (suggesting low sleep efficiency)? • (See the "How to compute sleep efficiency" handout)
NAPS	• What is the frequency of the patient's naps? • What is the average duration of the naps? • At what time of the day are the naps taken? • Is there a relationship between napping and the quantity and quality of sleep in the previous or following night?
SLEEP QUALITY	• Is there significant night-to-night variability in the patient's assessment of his or her sleep quality? • Is there a relationship between the patient's subjective sleep quality and other nighttime parameters (time awake, total sleep time, time spent in bed)?
SUBSTANCE USE	• Does the patient systematically use medication, alcohol, or drugs to help him or her fall asleep? • Does the patient believe that he or she will be able to sleep without these substances?

Clinician guide
How to Compute Sleep Efficiency

- Sleep efficiency is a very good indicator of sleep difficulties and **can be estimated using the sleep diary**. It is computed as follows:

$$\text{Sleep efficiency} = \frac{\text{Total sleep time}}{\text{Time spent in bed at night}} \times 100$$

- Sleep efficiency is the percentage of time spent in bed during which the individual is actually sleeping.

- Sleep efficiency can be calculated for a single night; however, since sleep can vary significantly from one night to another, it is preferable to compute it over a longer period, for example, 1 or 2 weeks. This yields a more accurate estimate of the individual's regular sleep.

- Sleep efficiency can be estimated based on general sleep habits. However, it is calculated more reliably using the sleep diary. See the following page for an example of how to calculate sleep efficiency for a single night.

- The average sleep efficiency over a longer period can easily be calculated by adding up sleep efficiency for all nights in this period and then dividing the sum by the number of nights. For example, average efficiency over a 1-week period can be found by adding up the sleep efficiency calculated for each of the 7 nights of the week, then dividing the total by seven (number of nights).

- Usually, people without sleep difficulties (good sleepers) have a sleep efficiency of 85% or greater, meaning that they sleep at least 85% of the time they spend in bed at night. This threshold is somewhat arbitrary, but it can be useful for comparison purposes.

- Higher sleep efficiency is generally an indication of better sleep quality, and more continuous, less interrupted sleep.

How to Compute Sleep Efficiency (example with the sleep diary)

ID: _____

		Date
		July 9, 2014
1.	Yesterday, I napped from _____ to _____. (record the times for all naps)	10:00-10:15 a.m. 12:30-4:00 p.m.
2.	I got into bed at _____. (record the time)	10:15 p.m.
3.	I tried to go to sleep at _____. (record the time)	10:30 p.m.
4.	After turning the lights off, it took me _____ to fall asleep.	15 min
5.	My sleep was interrupted _____ times. (record the number of awakenings)	2
6.	In total, my sleep was interrupted for _____. (record total duration for all awakenings)	1 hr 30 min
7.	Last night, I got out of bed _____ times. (record the number of times you got out of bed)	1
8.	This morning, my final awakening was at _____. (record the time of your final awakening without going back to sleep)	6:15
9.	This morning, I got out of bed at _____. (record the time)	7:00
10.	The quality of my sleep from last night was _____. (1 to 5; 1 = very bad; 5 = very good)	3
11.	Yesterday, I took _____ to help me sleep. (e.g., medication, alcohol, drug, and natural product)	Zopiclone 7.5 mg

(A) Calculate total time spent in bed at night
Amount of time between:
- The time you started trying to fall asleep .... 10:30 p.m.
  and
- The time you got out of bed .... 7:00 a.m.
  =
Time spent in bed: .... **8 hr 30 (510 min)**

(B) Calculate total time spent awake
Time needed to fall asleep .... 0 hr 15 min
  +
Total duration of awakenings .... 1 hr 30 min (90 min)
  +
Time between waking and getting out of bed (6:15 a.m. to 7 a.m.) .... 0 hr 45 min
  =
Time spent awake: .... **2 hr 30 min (150 min)**

(C) Calculate total sleep time
Time spent in bed (A) .... 8 hr 30 min (510 min)
  -
Time spent awake (B) .... 2 hr 30 min (150 min)
  =
Total sleep time: .... **6 hr 00 min (360 min)**

(D) Calculate sleep efficiency
Total sleep time (C) .... 360 min
  ÷
Time spent in bed (A) .... 510 min
  ×
100 100
  =
Sleep efficiency: **70.6%**

 Insomnia Severity Index (ISI)

ID: _____Date: _____

For each following question, please circle the number corresponding most accurately to your sleep pattern **in the last month.**

For the first three questions, please rate the **SEVERITY** of your sleep difficulties.

1. Difficulty falling asleep:

None	Mild	Moderate	Severe	Very severe
0	1	2	3	4

2. Difficulty staying asleep:

None	Mild	Moderate	Severe	Very severe
0	1	2	3	4

3. Problem waking up too early in the morning:

None	Mild	Moderate	Severe	Very severe
0	1	2	3	4

4. How **SATISFIED/DISSATISFIED** are you with your current sleep pattern?

Very satisfied	Satisfied	Neutral	Dissatisfied	Very dissatisfied
0	1	2	3	4

5. To what extent do you consider your sleep problem to **INTERFERE** with your daily functioning (e.g., fatigue, concentration, memory, and mood)?

Not at all	A little	Somewhat	Much	Very much
0	1	2	3	4

6. How **NOTICEABLE** to others do you think your sleep problem is in terms of impairing the quality of your life?

Not at all	A little	Somewhat	Much	Very much
0	1	2	3	4

7. How **WORRIED/DISTRESSED** are you about your current sleep problem?

Not at all	A little	Somewhat	Much	Very much
0	1	2	3	4

Source: From Morin, C. M. (1993). Treatment manuals for practitioners. Insomnia: Psychological assessment and management. Reprinted with permission of Guilford Press.

Clinician guide
Insomnia Severity Index (ISI)—Scoring and Interpretation

Scoring:
- Add up scores for questions 1–7 (total score ranging from 0 to 28).

Interpretation
- Categories:

0–7	No insomnia
8–14	Subthreshold insomnia
15–21	Moderate insomnia
22–28	Severe insomnia

- Threshold score: any score of more than 10 qualifies as a case of insomnia;

- An improvement of 8 points or more (e.g., between measurements taken before and after treatment for insomnia) is considered to be clinically significant.

For more information:

Morin, C. M. (1993). *Insomnia: Psychological assessment and management*. New York: Guilford.

Bastien, C. H., Vallières, A., & Morin, C. M. (2001). Validation of the Insomnia Severity Index as an outcome measure for insomnia research. *Sleep Medicine, 2*, 297–307.

Morin, C. M., Belleville, G., Bélanger, L., & Ivers, H. (2011). The Insomnia Severity Index: Psychometric indicators to detect insomnia cases and evaluate treatment response. *Sleep, 34*, 601–608.

Gagnon, C., Bélanger, L., Ivers, H., & Morin, C. M. (2013). Validation of the Insomnia Severity Index in primary care. *Journal of the American Board of Family Medicine, 26*, 701–710.

 Dysfunctional Beliefs and Attitudes about Sleep (DBAS)

ID: _____Date: _____

DYSFUNCTIONAL BELIEFS AND ATTITUDES ABOUT SLEEP (DBAS)
Several statements reflecting people's beliefs and attitudes about sleep are listed below. Please indicate to what extent you personally agree or disagree with each statement. There is no right or wrong answer. For each statement, circle the number that corresponds to your own **personal belief**. Please respond to all items even though some may not apply directly to your own situation.

Strongly disagree									Strongly agree
0	1	2	3	4	5	6	(7)	8	9	10

Source: *From Morin, C. M. (1993). Treatment manuals for practitioners. Insomnia: Psychological assessment and management. Reprinted with permission of Guilford Press.*

1. I need 8 hours of sleep to feel refreshed and function well during the day.

    0   1   2   3   4   5   6   7   8   9   10

2. When I don't get proper amount of sleep on a given night, I need to catch up on the next day by napping or on the next night by sleeping longer.

    0   1   2   3   4   5   6   7   8   9   10

3. Because I am getting older, I need less sleep.

    0   1   2   3   4   5   6   7   8   9   10

4. I am worried that if I go for 1 or 2 nights without sleep, I may have a "nervous breakdown."

    0   1   2   3   4   5   6   7   8   9   10

Strongly disagree										Strongly agree
0	1	2	3	4	5	6	7	8	9	10

5. I am concerned that chronic insomnia may have serious consequences on my physical health.

0	1	2	3	4	5	6	7	8	9	10

6. By spending more time in bed, I usually get more sleep and feel better the next day

0	1	2	3	4	5	6	7	8	9	10

7. When I have trouble falling asleep or getting back to sleep after nighttime awakening, I should stay in bed and try harder.

0	1	2	3	4	5	6	7	8	9	10

8. I am worried that I may lose control over my abilities to sleep.

0	1	2	3	4	5	6	7	8	9	10

9. Because I am getting older, I should go to bed earlier in the evening.

0	1	2	3	4	5	6	7	8	9	10

10. After a poor night's sleep, I know that it will interfere with my daily activities on the next day.

0	1	2	3	4	5	6	7	8	9	10

11. In order to be alert and function well during the day, I believe I would be better off taking a sleeping pill rather than having a poor night's sleep.

0	1	2	3	4	5	6	7	8	9	10

12. When I feel irritable, depressed, or anxious during the day, it is mostly because I did not sleep well the night before.

0	1	2	3	4	5	6	7	8	9	10

Strongly disagree										Strongly agree
0	1	2	3	4	5	6	7	8	9	10

13. Because my bed partner falls asleep as soon as his/her head hits the pillow and stays asleep through the night, I should be able to do so too.

0	1	2	3	4	5	6	7	8	9	10

14. I feel that insomnia is basically the result of aging, and there isn't much that can be done about this problem.

0	1	2	3	4	5	6	7	8	9	10

15. I am sometimes afraid of dying in my sleep.

0	1	2	3	4	5	6	7	8	9	10

16. When I have a good night's sleep, I know that I will have to pay for it on the following night.

0	1	2	3	4	5	6	7	8	9	10

17. When I sleep poorly on one night, I know it will disturb my sleep schedule for the whole week.

0	1	2	3	4	5	6	7	8	9	10

18. Without an adequate night's sleep, I can hardly function the next day.

0	1	2	3	4	5	6	7	8	9	10

19. I can't ever predict whether I'll have a good or poor night's sleep.

0	1	2	3	4	5	6	7	8	9	10

20. I have little ability to manage the negative consequences of disturbed sleep.

0	1	2	3	4	5	6	7	8	9	10

Strongly disagree										Strongly agree
0	1	2	3	4	5	6	7	8	9	10

21. When I feel tired, have no energy, or just seem not to function well during the day, it is generally because I did not sleep well the night before.

0	1	2	3	4	5	6	7	8	9	10

22. I get overwhelmed by my thoughts at night and often feel I have no control over this racing mind.

0	1	2	3	4	5	6	7	8	9	10

23. I feel I can still lead a satisfactory life despite sleep difficulties.

0	1	2	3	4	5	6	7	8	9	10

24. I believe insomnia is essentially the result of a chemical imbalance.

0	1	2	3	4	5	6	7	8	9	10

25. I feel insomnia is ruining my ability to enjoy life and preventing me from doing what I want.

0	1	2	3	4	5	6	7	8	9	10

26. A "nightcap" before bedtime is a good solution to a sleep problem.

0	1	2	3	4	5	6	7	8	9	10

27. Medication is probably the only solution to sleeplessness.

0	1	2	3	4	5	6	7	8	9	10

28. My sleep is getting worse all the time, and I don't believe anyone can help.

0	1	2	3	4	5	6	7	8	9	10

Strongly disagree										Strongly agree
0	1	2	3	4	5	6	7	8	9	10

29. It usually shows in my physical appearance when I haven't slept well.

0	1	2	3	4	5	6	7	8	9	10

30. I avoid or cancel obligations (social, family) after a poor night's sleep.

0	1	2	3	4	5	6	7	8	9	10

Clinician guide
Dysfunctional Beliefs and Attitudes about Sleep (DBAS)—Scoring and Interpretation

Scoring
- Calculate the average for answers to questions 1–30. (**Note:** The score for question 23 must be reversed by subtracting the circled number from 10.)

Interpretation
- A higher score indicates stronger adherence to beliefs and attitudes that contribute to insomnia;
- There is no validated threshold score.

Use and intervention
- The questionnaire can be very useful for identifying intervention targets (beliefs and attitudes to discuss with the patient);
- The questions can be grouped into themes to facilitate intervention:
  - Unrealistic expectations regarding sleep needs and daytime functioning (questions 1, 13, 16, 17);
  - Misattributions of the causes of insomnia (questions 3, 9, 14, 24);
  - Exaggerated perception of the consequences of insomnia (questions 5, 10, 12, 15, 18, 21, 23, 25, 29, 30);
  - Misconceptions regarding practices that are beneficial to sleep (questions 2, 6, 7, 11, 26, 27);
  - Excessive worrying and sense of loss of control (questions 4, 8, 19, 20, 22, 28).
- For some patients, it may be worthwhile to discuss elements that they strongly agreed with (e.g., above 5/10).

For more information:

Morin, C. M. (1993). *Insomnia: Psychological assessment and management*. New York: Guilford.

Carney, C. E., Edinger, J. D., Morin, C. M., Manber, R., Rybarczyk, B., Stepanksi, E. J., Wright, H., & Lack, L. (2010). Examining maladaptive beliefs about sleep across insomnia patient groups. *Journal of Psychosomatic Research, 68*, 57–65.

Morin, C. M., Vallières, A., & Ivers, H. (2007). Dysfunctional beliefs and attitudes about sleep: Validation of a brief version (DBAS-16). *Sleep, 30*, 1547–1554.

 Case Conceptualization Summary for Post-TBI Insomnia

NATURE AND SEVERITY OF INSOMNIA
EFFECTS OF INSOMNIA ON PERSONAL FUNCTIONING

PREDISPOSING FACTORS	PRECIPITATING FACTORS
MEDICAL FACTORS	ENVIRONMENTAL FACTORS

BEHAVIORAL PERPETUATING FACTORS (HABITS)

COGNITIVE PERPETUATING FACTORS (THOUGHTS/ATTITUDES/ BELIEFS/EXPECTATIONS)

NEUROPSYCHOLOGICAL OR BEHAVIORAL PARTICULARITIES

TREATMENT PLAN

Assessment Tools for Post-TBI Fatigue

OVERVIEW

This chapter is a compendium of assessment tools for post-TBI insomnia. It includes the following tools and clinician guides:

- Proposed diagnostic criteria for TBI-related fatigue
- Clinical interview on fatigue following traumatic brain injury
- Energy/Activity diary
- Energy/Activity diary—example and instructions
- Energy/Activity diary—analysis
- Multidimensional fatigue inventory (MFI)
- Fatigue severity scale (FSS)
- Fatigue numerical rating scale
- Fatigue barometer
- Case conceptualization summary for post-TBI fatigue

Clinician guide
Proposed Diagnostic Criteria for TBI-Related Fatigue

A. Significant fatigue, diminished energy, or increased need to rest, disproportionate to any recent change in activity level. This fatigue is present for more than half of the day, almost every day, and is associated with at least one of the following symptoms: - Complaints of generalized weakness or limb heaviness; - Diminished concentration, attention, or memory; - Decreased motivation or interest to engage in usual activities; - Perceived need to struggle to overcome inactivity; - Marked emotional reactivity (e.g., sadness, frustration, or irritability) to feeling fatigued; - Difficulty completing daily tasks attributed to feeling fatigued; - Perceived problems with short-term memory; - Postexertion malaise lasting several hours.
B. The fatigue lasts at least three months.
C. The symptoms are present for more than half of the day.
D. The symptoms cause clinically significant distress or impairment in social, occupational, or other important areas of functioning.
E. The symptoms decrease the quality of life.
F. There is evidence from the history, physical examination, or laboratory findings that the symptoms are a consequence of traumatic brain injury.
G. The symptoms are not primarily a consequence of comorbid psychiatric disorders such as major depression.
NOTE: In the absence of diagnostic criteria specific to post-TBI fatigue, we have proposed a combination of criteria from the following sources: Boiko, A. N. et al. (2007). Characteristics of the formation of chronic fatigue syndrome and approaches to its treatment in young patients with focal brain damage. *Neuroscience and Behavioral Physiology*, 37, 221−228. Cella, D. et al. (1998). Progress towards guidelines for the management of fatigue. *Oncology*, 12, 369−377.

 **Clinical Interview on Fatigue Following Traumatic Brain Injury**

Patient ID:	Date:

For this series of questions, think back over the past month.

1. How much fatigue have you been feeling lately? How would you describe your energy level?

   _____

2. How long have you been having fatigue-related problems?

   _____

3. Did you have fatigue-related problems before your ☐ Yes ☐ No
   TBI occurred?

   If so, did you need to interrupt your activities during
   the day to take a nap or rest before the accident? _____

4. How did your energy/fatigue evolve since the accident:
   During the acute phase/hospitalization:

   _____

   The first few weeks/months at home:

   _____

   When returning to your preinjury activities (family roles, work,
   studies, leisure, etc.):

   _____

5. How often do you feel fatigue over the course of a typical week?

Never	Rarely	A few times per week	Almost every day of the week	Every day of the week
0	1	2	3	4

6. How much fatigue do you feel at the following times of day (on a scale from 1 to 10, 1 = no fatigue, 10 = extreme fatigue)?

Morning upon waking	
Morning (general)	
Afternoon	
Dinnertime	
Evening	

7. During which part of day do you feel most energetic? _____

8. During which part of day do you feel most tired?_____

9. Do you need to interrupt your activities during the day in order to rest or to take a nap?   ☐ Yes   ☐ No

   If so, how often?_____

   Can you provide some examples: _____

   _____

10. What types of activities do you feel are most tiring, demanding (ask about physical and intellectual activities, daily tasks which may require concentration or planning)?

   _____

11. Do you take naps (actually sleeping) during the day?   ☐ Yes   ☐ No

   If so, how often? _____

   About how long are your naps?_____

   When in the day do you take your naps?_____

   How do you feel after a nap (very/slightly rested, equally/slightly more/much more tired)? _____

12. Do you take rest periods (without sleeping) during the day?   ☐ Yes   ☐ No

   If so, how often? _____

   How long are your rest periods? _____

   When in the day do you take your rest periods? _____

   How do you feel after a rest period (very/slightly rested, equally/slightly more/much more tired)? _____

13. How does fatigue affect your everyday life?

_____

_____

14. How much would you say that fatigue affects the following …

(1 = no effect/no impact, 10 = considerable effect/extreme impact)
 a) Your daily routine? _____

 b) Your mood? _____

 c) Your mental capacities (attention, concentration, and memory)? _____

 d) Your social or leisure activities?_____

 e) Your family or love life?_____

 f) Your main occupation (work, studies, or volunteering)? _____

 g) Other spheres of life?_____

15. How apparent do you think your fatigue is to other people in terms of a deterioration in your quality of life (1 = not at all apparent, 10 = extremely apparent)?

_____

16. How concerned or worried are you about your level of fatigue (1 = not at all concerned, 10 = extremely concerned)? _____

What worries you the most?

_____

17. What, in your opinion, is the cause of your fatigue (e.g., stress, pain, depression, medication, activities, nothing in particular)?

_____

18. What factors do you think aggravate your fatigue?

_____

19. Among the following, which elements apply to your situation and how much does each contribute to your energy level and fatigue during the day?

	Nature, frequency, and severity of difficulties	Do you think this contributes to your fatigue?
Anxiety, nervousness, and worrying		
Depression, sadness, and loss of interest		
Alcohol or drug use		
Pain		
Medical problem		
Use of prescribed or over-the-counter medication		

20. Are you physically active? What are your exercise habits?

_____

21. Do you wish to increase your physical activity level? What barriers or facilitators do you see relative to exercise?

_____

22. What strategies do you use when you want to deal with your fatigue? How are these working for you?

_____

_____

23. Have you reduced some activities, or do you avoid some activities because of your fatigue?

_____

_____

24. Do you think your fatigue affects the people around you? How so? Do people close to you sometimes help you because of your fatigue?

_____

_____

25. If you felt more energetic, which activities you would want to do more of?

_____

_____

Energy/Activity Diary

Rate your energy (or fatigue) level for each of the following times of day, using the scale below:

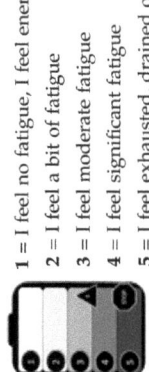

1 = I feel no fatigue, I feel energetic
2 = I feel a bit of fatigue
3 = I feel moderate fatigue
4 = I feel significant fatigue
5 = I feel exhausted, drained of energy

Take notes about activities, naps, rest periods, meal times, emotions, etc.

Date				
Bedtime last night				
Rising time this morning				
Upon waking up this morning - Level of fatigue (1 to 5) - Activities/Meals/Naps/Emotion				
Morning - Level of fatigue (1 to 5) - Activities/Meals/Naps/Emotion				
Afternoon - Level of fatigue (1 to 5) - Activities/Meals/Naps/Emotion				
Dinnertime - Level of fatigue (1 to 5) - Activities/Meals/Naps/Emotion				
Evening - Level of fatigue (1 to 5) - Activities/Meals/Naps/Emotion				

Adapted from the *Guide de l'énergie*, Institut de réadaptation en déficience physique de Québec.

HELPFUL SUGGESTIONS FOR EFFICIENT ENERGY MANAGEMENT

Engage in regular physical exercise (e.g., walk every day).

Maintain a healthy lifestyle (regular meals and regular sleep schedule).

Recognize your signs of fatigue. Keep track of which activities require more or less energy.

Plan more demanding activities with care:

- Choose a time of day when you feel more energetic;
- Make sure to alternate with less demanding tasks;
- Break down activities into manageable steps to avoid getting exhausted.

Adopt the following attitudes:

- Congratulate yourself for completing one step of a task, or part of an activity rather than being frustrated for not completing it;
- Accept help when possible;
- Do not avoid social occasions or pleasant activities because of fatigue, rather plan shorter or simpler activities so that you can benefit from these without getting exhausted.

WHAT DID I LEARN THIS WEEK ? WHAT COULD I DO DIFFERENTLY NEXT WEEK ?

_____

_____

_____

_____

_____

_____

_____

_____

_____

_____

_____

Adapted from the *Guide de l'énergie*, Institut de réadaptation en déficience physique de Québec.

Energy/Activity Diary—Example and Instructions

Date	Wednesday	→ Write down the day of the week.
Bedtime last night	10:30 p.m.	→ Write down the time you went to bed last night.
Rising time this morning	9:30 a.m.	→ Right down the time you got up.

Upon waking up this morning
- Level of fatigue (1 to 5)
- Activities/Meals/Naps/
  Emotions
	3
	
	Slept poorly
	back pain
	Difficulty moving
	
	Didn't have breakfast
		→ Rate your level of fatigue in the upper left-hand corner of each box using the following scale:
		  1 = I feel no fatigue, I feel energetic
		  2 = I feel slight fatigue
		  3 = I feel moderate fatigue
		  4 = I feel significant fatigue
		  5 = I feel exhausted, drained of energy

Morning - Level of fatigue (1 to 5) - Activities/Meals/Naps/ Emotions	**4** Cleaned up kitchen Tax papers 10 a.m.–1 p.m. Pizza Headache	→ Write down your activities, regardless of whether or not they seem related to fatigue. Also write down your symptoms and your meals.
Afternoon - Level of fatigue (1 to 5) - Activities/Meals/Naps/ Emotions	**5** Exhausted Slept from 1:30 to 3:40 p.m. Email	→ Write down your naps.
Suppertime - Level of fatigue (1 to 5) - Activities/Meals/Naps/ Emotions	**4** Didn't go to my sister's because I was too tired Soup, cheese	→ Write down any social or leisure activities you missed or declined because of fatigue.
Evening - Level of fatigue (1 to 5) - Activities/Meals/Naps/ Emotions	**3** television Disappointed because I didn't do much unable to finish filling out tax documents	→ Write down your emotions, impressions, or other relevant information.

Clinician guide
Energy/Activity Diary—Analysis

ACTIVITY PATTERNS	— Is the patient's activity schedule regular or fairly variable? — Do the frequency and nature of the reported activities seem adapted to the patient's reality or condition? — Are there long periods of inactivity during the day or over several days after a more intense activity (cycles of overexertion followed by much less active periods)? — Does the patient nap too frequently, for too long, or too late in the day? — Are naps or inactivity the patient's only means of rest?
LIFE STYLE	— Does the patient eat at fairly regular times? — Does the patient engage in physical exercise? — Does the patient have a fairly regular sleep schedule and satisfactory sleep? — Is the fatigue related to unhealthy lifestyle habits (heavy meals, alcohol or recreational drug consumption, or inactivity)?
TIRING ACTIVITIES	— Does the patient feel greater fatigue during activities that require mental effort (e.g., organization, concentration, memory, sustained social interactions) and/or physical exertion? — Is the fatigue greater following more stressful activities?
ENERGY-LEVEL FLUCTUATIONS	— Looking over several days, are there times of day when the patient feels more or less energetic? How does this relate to the patient's activities? — Are there days when the patient feels more energetic or more tired? How does this relate to the patient's activities? — Do you notice certain times (or risk situations) that are typically more difficult for the patient and that would require special attention?

 **Multidimensional Fatigue Inventory (MFI)**

Patient ID: _____Date: _____

Using the following statements, we would like to understand how you felt recently. For each statement, circle the appropriate number to the right of the statement. For instance, if you think a statement is entirely true, that you strongly agree, circle the number 5. Following is an example:

I feel rested .... 1 2 3 4 ⑤

Answer all questions by circling the appropriate number using the following scale:

1	2	3	4	5
Strongly disagree				Strongly agree

	Your answers
1. I feel fit.	1 2 3 4 5
2. Physically, I feel only able to do a little.	1 2 3 4 5
3. I feel very active.	1 2 3 4 5
4. I feel like doing all sorts of nice things.	1 2 3 4 5
5. I feel tired.	1 2 3 4 5
6. I think I do a lot in a day.	1 2 3 4 5
7. When I am doing something, I can keep my thoughts on it.	1 2 3 4 5
8. Physically, I can take on a lot.	1 2 3 4 5
9. I dread having to do things.	1 2 3 4 5
10. I think I do very little in a day.	1 2 3 4 5
11. I can concentrate well.	1 2 3 4 5
12. I am rested.	1 2 3 4 5
13. It takes a lot of effort to concentrate on things.	1 2 3 4 5
14. Physically, I feel I am in bad condition.	1 2 3 4 5
15. I have a lot of plans.	1 2 3 4 5
16. I tire easily.	1 2 3 4 5
17. I get little done.	1 2 3 4 5
18. I don't feel like doing anything.	1 2 3 4 5
19. My thoughts easily wander.	1 2 3 4 5
20. Physically, I feel I am in excellent condition.	1 2 3 4 5

Clinician guide
Multidimensional Fatigue Inventory (MFI)—Scoring and Interpretation

Scoring:
- The inventory is made up of five subscales, each of which includes four questions: two positively and two negatively worded (identified with *):
  - General Fatigue (items 1*, 5, 12*, 16)
  - Physical fatigue (items 2, 8*, 14, 20*)
  - Mental Fatigue (items 7*, 11*, 13, 19)
  - Reduced Activities (items 3*, 6*, 10, 17)
  - Reduced Motivation (items 4*, 9, 15*, 18)
- A total of 10 of the 20 items (items 1, 3, 4, 6, 7, 8, 11, 12, 15 and 20) need to be inverted (answer subtracted from 6);
  - 1 becomes 5
  - 2 becomes 4
  - 3 becomes 3
  - 4 becomes 2
  - 5 becomes 1
- To obtain total subscale scores, the scores for the items of each subscale must be added together (total score minimum = 4; maximum = 20 with higher scores indicating greater fatigue levels).

Interpretation:
- No interpretation scales are provided by the authors of the questionnaire, and no Canadian or American epidemiological data is available;
- Age- and gender-based threshold scores have been suggested for the subscale of general fatigue according to German epidemiological data (Schwarz et al., 2003; Singer et al., 2011). These scores correspond to the 25th percentile of the German population.

Threshold scores suggesting the presence of significant fatigue (subscale of general fatigue only)			
	≤ 39 years old	40−59 years old	≥ 60 years old
Men	≥ 9	≥ 11	≥ 14
Women	≥ 11	≥ 12	≥ 14

For more information:

Smets, E. M., Garssen, B., Bonke, B., & De Haes, J. C. (1995). The Multidimensional Fatigue Inventory (MFI): Psychometric qualities of an instrument to assess fatigue. *Journal of Psychosomatic Research*, 39, 315–325.

Singer, S. et al. (2011). Age- and sex-standardised prevalence rates of fatigue in a large hospital-based sample of cancer patients. *British Journal of Cancer*, 105, 445–451.

Schwarz, R., Krauss, O., & Hinz, A. (2003). Fatigue in the general population. *Onkologie*, 26, 140–144.

Beaulieu-Bonneau, S., & Morin, C. M. (2012). Sleepiness and fatigue following traumatic brain injury. *Sleep Medicine, 13*, 598–605.

Beaulieu-Bonneau S. & Ouellet M-C. (2107). Fatigue in the first year after traumatic brain injury: course, relationship with injury severity, and correlates. *Neuropsychological Rehabilitation, 27*, 983–1001.

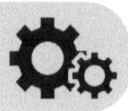 **Fatigue Severity Scale (FSS)**

Patient ID:_____Date:_____

Please circle the number between 1 and 7 which you feel best fits the following statements. This refers to your usual way of life within the last week. 1 indicates "strongly disagree" and 7 indicates "strongly agree."

Read and circle a number.	*Strongly Disagree (1) →* *Strongly Agree (7)*
1. My motivation is lower when I am fatigued.	1 2 3 4 5 6 7
2. Exercise brings on my fatigue.	1 2 3 4 5 6 7
3. I am easily fatigued.	1 2 3 4 5 6 7
4. Fatigue interferes with my physical functioning.	1 2 3 4 5 6 7
5. Fatigue causes frequent problems for me.	1 2 3 4 5 6 7
6. My fatigue prevents sustained physical functioning.	1 2 3 4 5 6 7
7. Fatigue interferes with carrying out certain duties and responsibilities.	1 2 3 4 5 6 7
8. Fatigue is among my most disabling symptoms.	1 2 3 4 5 6 7
9. Fatigue interferes with my work, family, or social life	1 2 3 4 5 6 7

Source: *Reproduced with permission from Krupp L.B., LaRocca N.G., Muir-Nash J., & Steinberg A.D. (1989). The fatigue severity scale. Application to patients with multiple sclerosis and systemic lupus erythematosus. Arch Neurol, 46, 1121–3. Copyright © 1989 American Medical Association.*

Clinician guide
Fatigue Severity Scale (FSS)—Scoring and Interpretation

Scoring
- The scale has nine items. Scores for each item are added up for a total score. An average item score can also be calculated (total divided by 9)
- Minimum score = 9
- Maximum score = 63
- Higher scores indicate greater fatigue severity

Interpretation
- No data specific to TBI is available
- Krupp et al. (1989) proposed that a total score over 36 (average item score 4.0) is indicative of severe fatigue or need of a more thorough evaluation in a population of persons with multiple sclerosis and systematic lupus erythematosus (mean age 40 years)
- Valko et al. (2008) calculated the mean of individual scores (total score divided by 9) and found the following mean scores for different groups of patients and healthy controls:

Group	Mean FSS score, standard deviation, (% with score ≥ 4.0)
Multiple sclerosis	4.66 ± 1.64 (69% with scores ≥ 4.0)
Previous ischemic stroke	3.90 ± 1.85 (49% with scores ≥ 4.0)
Sleep—wake disorders	4.34 ± 1.64 (62% with scores ≥ 4.0)
Healthy controls	3.00 ± 1.08 (18% with scores ≥ 4.0)

For more information:
Krupp L.B., LaRocca N.G., Muir-Nash J., & Steinberg A.D. (1989). The fatigue severity scale. Application to patients with multiple sclerosis and systemic lupus erythematosus. Arch Neurol, 46, 1121–3.

Valko P.O., Bassetti, C. L. Bloch, K. E. Held, U. &Baumann, C.R. (2008). Validation of the Fatigue Severity Scale in a Swiss Cohort. Sleep, 31, 1601–1607.

https://www.sralab.org/rehabilitation-measures/fatigue-severity-scale.

 **Fatigue Numerical Rating Scale**

Patient ID:_____

Use the following scale to rate the level of fatigue (from 0 to 10) you experience at different times during the same day or on different days. Note your activities.

Date, time: _____
Activity: _____

0	1	2	3	4	5	6	7	8	9	10
No fatigue			Slight fatigue				Moderate fatigue			Severe fatigue

---

Date, time: _____
Activity: _____

0	1	2	3	4	5	6	7	8	9	10
No fatigue			Slight fatigue				Moderate fatigue			Severe fatigue

---

Date, time: _____
Activity: _____

0	1	2	3	4	5	6	7	8	9	10
No fatigue			Slight fatigue				Moderate fatigue			Severe fatigue

---

Date, time: _____
Activity: _____

0	1	2	3	4	5	6	7	8	9	10
No fatigue			Slight fatigue				Moderate fatigue			Severe fatigue

---

Fatigue Barometer

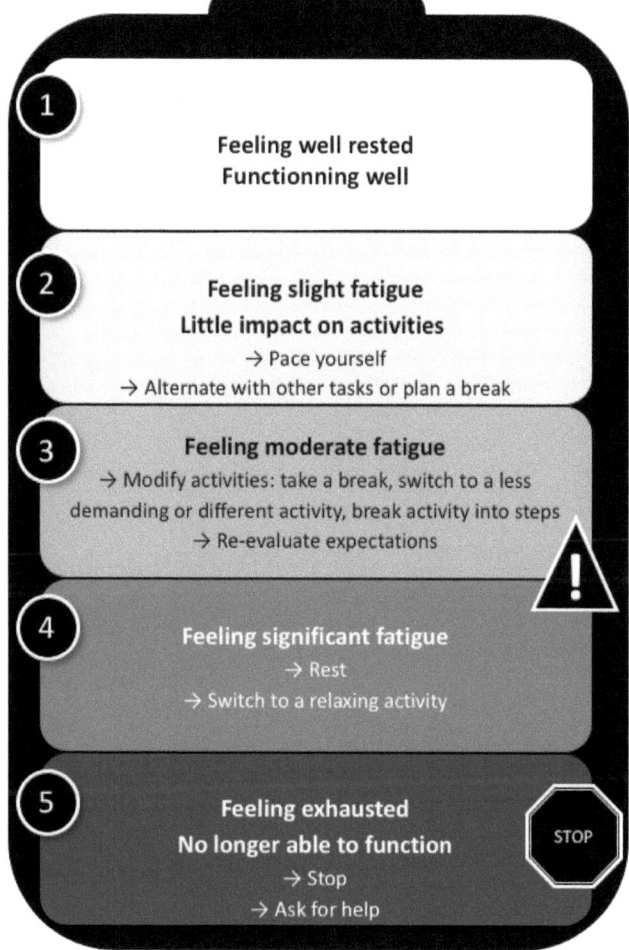

 Case Conceptualization Summary for Post-TBI Fatigue

NATURE AND SEVERITY OF FATIGUE
EFFECTS OF FATIGUE ON PERSONAL FUNCTIONING

PREDISPOSING FACTORS	PRECIPITATING FACTORS
MEDICAL FACTORS	ENVIRONMENTAL FACTORS

BEHAVIORAL PERPETUATING FACTORS (HABITS)

COGNITIVE PERPETUATING FACTORS (THOUGHTS/ATTITUDES/BELIEFS/EXPECTATIONS)

NEUROPSYCHOLOGICAL OR BEHAVIORAL PARTICULARITIES

TREATMENT PLAN

6

Intervention Tools for Post-TBI Insomnia

OVERVIEW

This chapter is a compendium of intervention tools for post-TBI insomnia. These tools should be used with a thorough understanding of their evidence base, rationale, and procedures, and after an exhaustive evaluation. It is therefore important to refer to Chapters 1 to 5 to ensure adequate preparation for intervention. This chapter includes the following Clinician Guides and corresponding handouts for patients:

Clinician Guides	Patient Handouts
• Overview of interventions strategies for post-TBI insomnia	• Self-management of insomnia • Helping a family member or friend manage insomnia (for significant others)
• Establishing effective self-monitoring with the sleep diary	• An essential tool: the sleep diary
• Presenting basic information on insomnia	• Sleep following a traumatic brain injury • What is chronic insomnia and how common is it? • What causes insomnia? • Factors which perpetuate insomnia
• Presenting basic information on sleep	• How sleep is produced • Stages of sleep and sleep cycles
• Presenting basic information on sleep hygiene	• Sleep hygiene: maintaining lifestyle habits that promote good sleep
• Stimulus control: Recreating a time and place for sleep	• Recreating a time and place for sleep
• Restriction of time in bed: Limiting the time spent in bed to actual sleeping time	• Limiting the time spent in bed to actual sleeping time
• Brief cognitive therapy: Promoting beliefs and attitudes that are conducive to sleep and managing worries	• Beliefs and attitudes that promote good sleep • Strategies for better management of worries when going to bed or during nighttime awakenings
• Motivational strategies when encountering resistance	
• Clinical challenges and solutions to adapt CBT to the context of TBI	

Clinician guide
Overview of Intervention Strategies for Post-TBI Insomnia

	Interventions	Goals
PSYCHOEDUCATION	**Introducing the self-management approach**	• To reinforce patient self-efficacy
	Establishing self-monitoring with the sleep diary	• To identify sleep difficulties and associated behaviors • To facilitate the implementation of behavioral strategies • To keep track of progress
	Presenting basic information on sleep and insomnia	• To provide the patient with basic concepts about sleep in general, how TBI affects sleep, and how insomnia develops • To normalize the patient's experiences and validate subjective experiences
	Presenting basic information on sleep hygiene	• To provide recommendations concerning the effects of environmental and lifestyle-related factors on sleep
COGNITIVE-BEHAVIORAL INTERVENTIONS	**Recreating a time and place for sleep (stimulus control)**	• To reinforce associations between sleep, the sleep period, and the sleep environment • To allow sleep to come when needed
	Limiting the time spent in bed to actual sleeping time (restriction of time in bed)	• To consolidate sleep over a shorter period • To decrease the fragmentation of sleep and promote deeper sleep • To allow sleep to come when needed
	Promoting beliefs and attitudes that are conducive to sleep and managing worries (brief cognitive therapy)	• To maintain realistic attitudes toward sleep • To become aware that insomnia has multiple causes • To avoid assigning daytime difficulties to a lack of sleep • To develop tolerance to the effects of an acute lack of sleep • To suggest strategies for managing worries in the evening and at night

NOTE: Chapter 8 presents an eight-session protocol which was evaluated in a clinical case series integrating intervention for both insomnia and fatigue (Ouellet & Morin, 2007, Archives of Physical Medicine and Rehabilitation, 88(12):1581−1592).

 Self-Management of Insomnia

During this intervention, you will develop personal management skills to start changing behaviors, attitudes, beliefs, and lifestyles which might be contributing to your sleep problem. This intervention is unlikely to eliminate completely your insomnia, but you will learn to manage your sleep and energy more effectively so that you can maintain a good quality of life and engage in the important activities in your life with satisfaction. Here are a few key ingredients for success with this approach:

➤ *Commit and work at it*
   Make working on your sleep–wake habits a priority during this intervention. The intervention does require effort and consistency, but you are ready to start.

➤ *Give yourself time*
   Do not expect results within a week or two. The pace of your improvement will vary depending on the nature and severity of your insomnia or fatigue, the presence of other physical or psychological problems, and your own motivation and efforts to apply the strategies.

➤ *Obtain the support of those close to you and share the rationale of the interventions*
   Asking for the support of your family/friends will help facilitate your improvement. All through the intervention, discuss why and how you are changing your habits with your loved ones so that they can encourage you. For example, you may have to explain to your significant other why you will be going to bed later, or why you will be getting up at night.

➤ *Maintain realistic expectations*
   Unrealistic expectations can lead to frustration and disappointment. Set achievable goals and have a discussion with your therapist or health-care provider when you have difficulty applying a recommendation or feel stuck.

➤ *Avoid comparing yourself with before the accident*

Constantly trying to "get back to how I was before" can create strong pressure that may be detrimental to your efforts. Instead, try to think about what would be an adequate night of sleep most of the time or an acceptable energy level given your current circumstances. Instead of looking back, look forward at the progress you make every day.

➤ *Maintain a scientific attitude*

Before concluding that the intervention and recommendations do not work for you, be sure to test them out thoroughly for at least a few weeks. The patients who show the most progress are those who thoroughly apply the recommendations consistently.

 **Helping a Family Member or Friend Manage Insomnia**

Insomnia is very common following a traumatic brain injury. Your family member or friend is in the process of developing personal management skills in order to change some behaviors, attitudes, and lifestyles that may be interfering with his or her sleep. This intervention is unlikely to completely eliminate insomnia. The goal of intervention is rather to learn to effectively manage sleep—wake behaviors in order to maintain a good quality of life. Some strategies may appear counterintuitive to you, for example, spending less time in bed or getting up during the night. Do not hesitate to communicate with your loved one's health-care provider if you need some explanations regarding this intervention.

What you can do to help your family member or friend:

✓ Be encouraging! Taking charge of managing insomnia requires effort and discipline. Encourage your family member or friend to apply the suggested strategies and remind him or her that several weeks might be needed before noticeable improvement occurs.

✓ Avoid viewing your family member or friend's fatigue as laziness or a lack of willpower. Fatigue and insomnia can be very incapacitating problems following a traumatic brain injury, and they are difficult to manage.

✓ Help establish sleep-friendly habits and environments: the bedroom should be calm, comfortable, and reserved for sleep (and sexual activities).

✓ Help establish a regular sleep—wake schedule, healthy eating habits, and relatively regular meal and activity times.

✓ Your family member or friend will possibly spend less time in bed, or even get up more frequently during the night at the beginning of the intervention. This is a normal part of the intervention process. Indeed, the goal is that the time spent in bed at night should correspond more closely with the time spent actually sleeping.

✓ The first few weeks of this intervention may be difficult for your loved one and his or her fatigue or sleepiness may increase at first. Again this is a normal effect of the intervention.

✓ If you currently sleep in the same bed, be flexible toward sleeping arrangements if your own sleep is affected during the beginning of the intervention (e.g., temporarily sleeping separately).

✓ Encourage your family member or friend to engage in regular physical exercise (but not too close to bedtime), which helps improve energy level, sleep, and mood.

✓ Encourage him or her to stay active, while respecting his or her personal rhythms and capacities. Naps and rest periods are not the only solutions to a lack of sleep or energy. You might also suggest alternative activities that can renew energy or just refresh the mind, such as social, enjoyable, or fulfilling activities.

✓ As much as possible, avoid indefinitely handling tasks that seem too exhausting for your family member or friend. By doing so, you will help him or her to gradually learn to resume these tasks through better energy management.

✓ Avoid jumping to the conclusion that your friend or family member's behavior is due to insomnia or fatigue if he or she is irritable, exhibits organization problems, struggles with his or her concentration or memory, or is aggressive. Many other factors might also be involved.

Clinician guide
Establishing Effective Self-Monitoring With the Sleep
Diary

Rationale and benefits of using the sleep diary

Restores the patient's sense of control over his or her sleep	➤ By enabling observation of sleep habits ➤ By identifying certain behavior patterns ➤ By identifying circumstances and factors associated with a poor night of sleep ➤ By providing emotional distance from problems ➤ By allowing the patient to consider changes to his or her habits
Gives the patient an active role in managing his or her sleep	➤ By allowing the patient to begin to structure his or her own time, after having been cared for during an acute care or rehabilitation but before returning home ➤ By allowing the patient to begin to implement self-management behaviors
Documents sleep difficulties	➤ By describing the severity and frequency of sleep difficulties ➤ By providing greater perspective (in spite of the insomnia, are there nights when the patient does sleep well?)
Helps treat sleep difficulties	➤ By identifying targets for treatment ➤ By enabling the application of certain techniques (changing sleep-related habits, establishing a regular schedule, etc.)
Evaluates progress	➤ By observing the progression of time spent awake, time spent sleeping, and sleep efficiency and by providing reinforcement for improvements

How to use the sleep diary effectively

➤ This manual contains two versions of the sleep diary. Choose the version of the diary that is best suited for the patient. The longer version is ideal as it contains more information but the abridged version may be more suitable for patients with greater cognitive difficulty or lower motivation level.

➤ Seeing all the days of the week at one glance is very useful for the therapist as this allows the detection of patterns or habits more easily.

➤ Irrespective of the version that is used, the patient should complete all sleep diary questions on a daily basis for at least 1 or 2 weeks before starting the intervention.

Take the time to demonstrate how to fill out the sleep diary

➤ Explain the sections of the diary, what needs to be written down. It can be helpful to practice filling out the sleep diary directly during the session by asking the patient to write down the information about his or her previous night.

➤ Show the patient the completed example and encourage him or her to refer to it as needed.

➤ Advise the patient that ideally all the questions should be answered and to avoid overly vague answers (e.g., "I didn't sleep all night").

➤ Emphasize that the idea is not to give exact times but to provide his or her best estimates. The patient does not need to check the exact time to answer the diary questions. In fact, it is strongly recommended not to look at the clock during the night, in order to avoid interfering with sleep.

➤ Encourage the patient to fill out the diary immediately after getting up in the morning, as details can be rapidly forgotten once the day starts.

➤ Suggest that the patient keep the sleep diary (and a pen) at his or her bedside, or in the bathroom, where it will be visible in the morning when waking up.

Analyze the diary in collaboration with the patient each week

➤ Ideally, the sleep diary should be used throughout the intervention.

➤ Each week, it is important to take a few minutes to analyze the diary with the patient (see Sleep diary—Analysis in the chapter on Assessing).

Suggest solutions to help the patient overcome difficulties

➤ Make sure the patient understands the importance and usefulness of filling out the sleep diary.

➤ If the patient exhibits resistance, use a motivational approach. Rather than being prescriptive, ask the patient what he or she would be willing to do over the following days and show empathy for the fact that the diary can require effort or be a burden.

➤ If the patient often forgets to fill out the diary, make sure it is visible in his or her environment (e.g., on a night stand, in the washroom). You may also suggest that the patient combine the sleep diary with a daily activity (e.g., filling it out while having breakfast in the morning).

➤ If it may help encourage adherence, the patient can use a smartphone to help with note-taking or schedule a reminder to fill out the diary.

➤ Provide an electronic version of the diary if it is easier for the patient to fill out (an electronic version is available in the companion website). Some free smartphone applications can be used as a sleep diary.

➤ If the patient prefers to use his or her own electronic or paper diary or an application, it is important to ensure that it contains the same key information as the sleep diary so that the clinician and patient can analyze the information, calculate sleep efficiency, and still observe patterns of behavior over time.

 An Essential Tool: The Sleep Diary

Learning to monitor your sleep by taking a few notes each day is a very important part of this intervention. Monitoring your sleep with a sleep diary will help you as follows:

- ✓ **To observe your sleep patterns**
- ✓ **To gain a sense of control over your sleep–wake patterns**
- ✓ **To understand what habits you can change**
- ✓ **To evaluate your progress throughout the intervention**

Use your sleep diary every day during the intervention.

Sleep Diary (Full Version)—Example and Instructions

ID : _____

		Date		
		July 9	→	Record the date the night ended (morning).
1.	Yesterday, I napped from ____ to ____ (record the times for all naps)	10 – 10:15 a.m. 3:30 – 4 p.m.	→	Record the start time and end time of all naps, even if unintentional (e.g., falling asleep in front of the TV).
2.	I got into bed at ____. (record the time)	10:15 p.m.	→	Record the time you went to bed.
3.	I tried to go to sleep at ____. (record the time)	10:30 p.m.	→	Record the time when you tried to go to sleep (can be identical to or different from bedtime).
4.	After turning the lights off, it took me ____ minutes to fall asleep.	15 min	→	Give your best estimate of the time you took to fall asleep after you began trying to do so.
5.	My sleep was interrupted ____ times. (record the number of awakenings)	2	→	Estimate the number of times you woke up during the night.
6.	In total, my sleep was interrupted for ____ minutes. (record the total duration for all awakenings)	1 hr 30 min	→	Estimate how much time you spent awake in total for all the times you woke up. Do not include your final awakening.
7.	Last night, I got out of bed ____ times. (record the number of times you got out of bed)	1	→	Record the number of times you got out of bed during the night.
8.	This morning, my final awakening was at ____. (record the time of your final awakening without going back to sleep)	6:15 a.m.	→	Record the final time you woke up without going back to sleep.
9.	This morning, I got out of bed at ____. (record the time)	7:00 a.m.	→	Record the time you got out of bed for the day.
10.	The quality of my sleep from last night was ____. (1 to 5; 1 = very bad; 5 = very good)	3	→	Estimate the overall quality of your sleep on a scale from 1–5.
11.	Yesterday, I took ____ to help me sleep: (e.g., medication, alcohol, drug, natural product)	Zopiclone 7.5 mg	→	Record any medication or substances you used to help you fall sleep last night.

Clinician guide
Presenting Basic Information on Insomnia

Rationale

➤ To normalize his or her experience.

➤ To help the patient clearly understand insomnia in order to be able to better distinguish it from other sleep problems.

➤ To make sure the patient understands that insomnia has multiple causes and that it is thus not caused exclusively by the brain injury.

➤ To make the patient aware that regardless of what led to the appearance or worsening of insomnia, several factors perpetuate insomnia over the long term and can be worked on in order to improve sleep.

Implementation in brief

Three topics will be addressed with the patient using the tools in the following pages:

➤ A general definition of insomnia

➤ The factors behind insomnia

➤ The influence of factors that perpetuate insomnia

It can be helpful to give the following handouts to the patient and to read and discuss them together, especially if the patient is interested in learning more about sleep. This information is not absolutely essential to the intervention's success, but it can boost patient motivation and commitment. If the patient has important cognitive issues, the first handout might suffice, the important message being that many factors influence sleep and contribute to insomnia, and that several of these can be modified.

Sleep Following a Traumatic Brain Injury

If you have sleep problems, you are not alone. Almost half of the patients with brain injury report difficulty in sleeping after their injury. Insomnia problems are especially frequent, whether in the form of difficulty in falling asleep, staying asleep, or getting restorative sleep. In the first few days or weeks after the accident, you probably spontaneously slept more than usual. For the majority of people, sleep tends to go back to normal. However, in some cases, sleep difficulties that began or worsened following a brain injury can become chronic. Although the brain injury may have affected your sleep, it is important to remember that a wide variety of other factors can influence sleep.

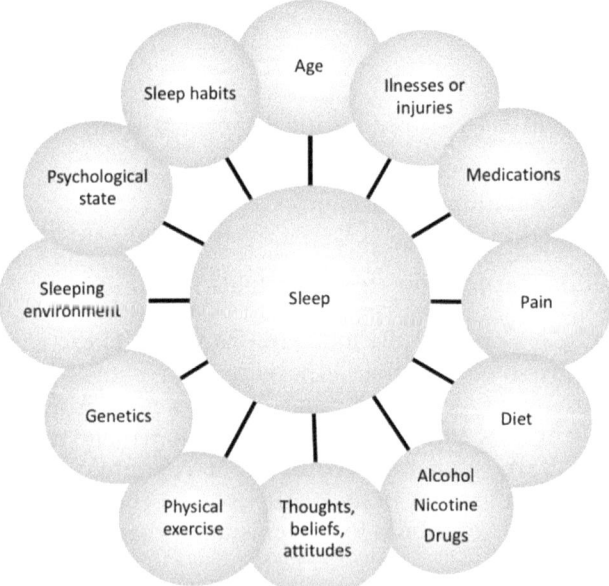

> Physical, psychological, and environmental factors can all influence sleep quality and quantity. Although some factors cannot be changed, others are modifiable with changes in lifestyle, behaviors, and ways of thinking.

What is Chronic Insomnia and How Common Is It?

What is chronic insomnia?	➢ It is characterized by a dissatisfaction with the quality or quantity of one's sleep.
	➢ Presenting/reporting one or more of the following symptoms:
	  - Difficulties falling asleep: taking more than 30 minutes to fall asleep.
	  - Frequent or prolonged nighttime awakenings: total awakening time of more than 30 minutes per night.
	  - Waking up too early in the morning: spontaneously waking up more than 30 minutes before the desired time.
	➢ The symptoms must be present at least three nights per week.
	➢ The insomnia must have been present for at least 3 months.
	➢ The insomnia must cause significant concern or distress, or adversely impact personal, social, family, or professional functioning.

What are the risk factors?	➢ Insomnia is more frequent in women than in men. ➢ Persons aged 60 and above are more prone to insomnia, not because of their age per se, but because of the changes that come with aging (change of roles, health issues, etc.). ➢ Persons with a medical (e.g., cancer), neurological (e.g., TBI), or psychological (e.g., major depression) medical condition are more vulnerable to insomnia regardless of their age.
How common is it?	➢ In the general population, roughly 30% of people have occasional sleep difficulties and 5–10% have chronic insomnia. ➢ Among individuals with traumatic brain injury, up to 50% have occasional sleep difficulties and up to 30% meet the criteria for chronic insomnia. ➢ Insomnia can occur after a mild traumatic brain injury just as well as after a moderate or severe injury.

 What Causes Insomnia?

Insomnia after TBI may be caused by a variety of factors, some that pre-dispose a person to insomnia in general, others that precipitate the sleep problem, and others that are known to maintain or perpetuate insomnia. Here are some examples of predisposing, precipitating, and perpetuating factors which may all contribute to cause insomnia.

Predisposing factors	➤ Consist of a person's biological or psychological characteristics. ➤ Are relatively stable over time, and difficult to change or control. ➤ Examples: Being a woman, being aged 60 or above, having a personal or family history of insomnia, or having an anxious or perfectionistic personality.
Precipitating factors	➤ Consist of a specific event or special circumstances that can trigger sleep difficulties. ➤ Sleep may get back to normal once the precipitating factor has disappeared or the patient has gotten used to it. When insomnia continues, while it can still be related to the residual effects of the precipitating factor, it is mainly due to the influence of perpetuating factors. ➤ Examples: Being sick, experiencing an injury, having pain, experiencing a stressful life event or period, for example, the death of a family member or friend, a new job, a separation, the birth of a child, financial difficulties, a hospitalization, a change of career path.
Perpetuating factors	➤ Consist of behaviors, habits, beliefs, and attitudes developed in response to insomnia. ➤ Instead of solving the problem, these factors contribute to maintain insomnia. ➤ These factors can be modified or controlled. Unlike the predisposing and most precipitating factors, they can be worked on in order to improve sleep. ➤ Examples: Taking long or frequent naps, having an irregular sleep schedule, watching television in bed, worrying about not getting enough sleep, going to bed too early, canceling appointments or activities to recuperate, etc.

Factors Which Perpetuate Insomnia

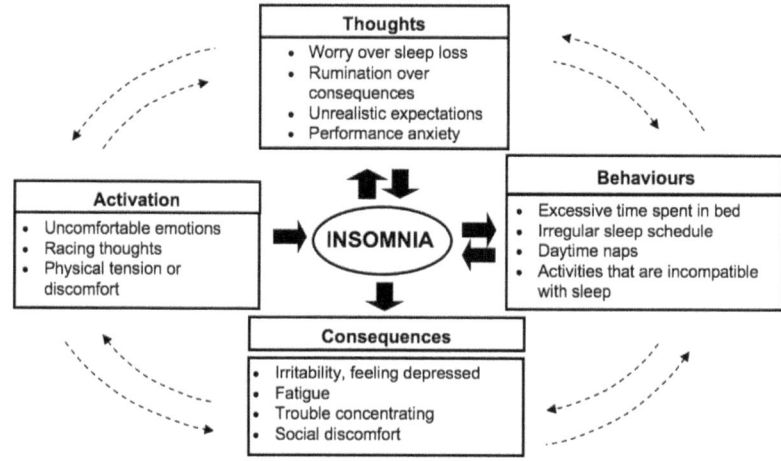

Source: *From Morin, C. M. (1993). Treatment manuals for practitioners. Insomnia: Psychological assessment and management. Reprinted with permission of Guilford Press.*

How to read this figure:

Activation	➤ This is often the starting point of an insomnia episode and can happen beginning, middle, or end of the night.
	➤ Activation is an emotional (stress, frustration), cognitive (racing thoughts), and/or physiological (pain, muscular tension) state that makes it difficult to fall asleep, or fall back asleep.
Behaviors	➤ When we do not sleep well, it is natural to try to make up for a lack of sleep or to try to sleep better. One might go to bed earlier, take a long nap in the afternoon, or cancel an activity. In the short term, these strategies could be useful. However, if they are used on the long term, these strategies may in fact be maintaining the insomnia problem—this program will show you why.
	➤ Behaviors, such as taking naps, irregular sleep—wake schedules, or using the bedroom for activities that are incompatible with sleep (e.g., watching TV or working on the computer in bed), are not necessarily detrimental for people without sleep difficulties. For people with insomnia, however, these behaviors may contribute to the problem.

Thoughts	➤ A number of attitudes (e.g., being overly concerned with insomnia) and beliefs about sleep or insomnia can increase anxiety about sleep. Being anxious about sleep is of course not very helpful. This program will teach you strategies to take some of this pressure off and let your body tell you when it is ready for sleep.
	➤ Having expectations that are unrealistic can make you feel rather helpless. This feeling exacerbates insomnia instead of helping to resolve it. Sleep is variable and influenced by many factors.
Consequences	➤ Of course, having a bad night of sleep can have negative consequences on daily functioning.
	➤ Sometimes, however, the consequences we feel contribute to our poor habits. For example, a person feeling tired or sleepy during the afternoon might decide to take a nap or go to bed much earlier. These behaviors in fact perpetuate insomnia.

Exercise:

Now look back on the figure and its explanation. Can you identify certain elements that fit with your own experience?

Clinician guide
Presenting Basic Information on Sleep

Rationale
➤ To validate the patient's subjective experience.
➤ To allow the patient to recognize the progression of a typical night of sleep.

Implementation in brief
Two topics will be addressed with the patient using the tools presented in the following pages:

➤ How sleep is produced
➤ Types of sleep and the sleep—wake cycle

This theoretical information is optional and not essential to the intervention's success. However, it can be useful for patients who wish to learn more about sleep. It can also reinforce patients' motivation to apply certain behavioral recommendations or help them understand and normalize certain sensations experienced during the night or day. For example, knowing that it is normal to perceive sleep as being lighter at the end of the night as opposed to the beginning of the night can be instructive for certain patients. They might then be more tolerant and worry less when they have early morning awakenings. Another example is knowing that it is natural for many people to feel slightly sleepier in the afternoon.

 ## How Sleep is Produced

The alternation between periods of wakefulness and sleep is regulated by the biological or circadian clock, which is located in our brain. Generally speaking, sleep is produced by two important factors, namely, the sleep drive and the biological clock.

Sleep drive	➤ The longer you are awake, the greater your tendency will be to fall asleep quickly and for a long time. For example, it is generally easier to fall asleep at night after 15 hours of being awake, as opposed to early in the morning after 2 hours of being awake.
	➤ Sleep drive is also responsible for the fact that several shorter nights of sleep will necessarily be followed by a longer night of good sleep.
	➤ In this intervention the proposed strategies will help you to maintain a healthy sleep drive each night at bedtime.
	➤ People with a healthy sleep drive usually have these habits: the time they spend in bed is about the same as the time they spend actually sleeping, they avoid naps, and, as much as possible, they get up and go to bed at the same time each day, even on weekends. These habits ensure that they actually feel sleepy by bedtime and fall asleep relatively easily.
Biological clock	➤ The brain synchronizes several bodily functions, such as our body temperature and the sleep—wake cycle, on a roughly 24-hour cycle.
	➤ The biological clock is sensitive to light (especially natural sunlight but also artificial light) and regular routines (meal times, periods of activity and inactivity). This is why having regular habits help maintain healthy sleep.
	➤ Generally speaking, the biological clock tends to keep people awake during the day and asleep at night.
	➤ During the day, all human beings experience certain low points when sleepiness is greater, and when mental capacities (attention, concentration, etc.) are weaker. This is the case in the early afternoon (around 2 p.m.) and at the end of the night (around 4 a.m.).

➤ One of the aims of this intervention will be to regulate your biological clock so that periods of wakefulness and sleep happen when needed.

➤ Here are few habits which help regulate the biological clock: get out of bed and go to bed at regular times, keep a regular work/activity or meal schedule, and expose yourself to sunlight early in the day while limiting light exposure in the evening.

Stages of Sleep and Sleep Cycles

- In a typical night, a person will go through different stages of sleep.

- A sleep cycle over a typical night is characterized by gradually going from light sleep (stages N1 and N2) to deep sleep (stage N3), then going back to lighter sleep stages (N1 and N2) before entering rapid eye movement sleep (or REM sleep). This stage is often closely linked to dreaming: if you are awakened during a REM sleep episode, you might remember being dreaming.

- One night will generally contain four to five of these sleep cycles.

- Deep sleep (N3) mainly occurs at the beginning of the night, thus, toward the end of the night, we spend more time in light sleep stages. REM sleep mainly occurs at the end of the night.

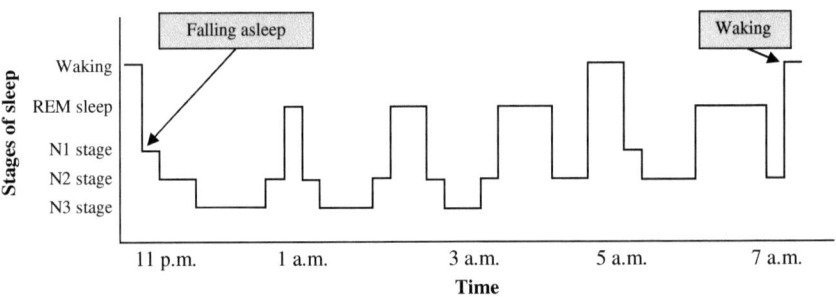

Clinician guide
Presenting Basic Information on Sleep Hygiene

Rationale

➤ To inform the patient about lifestyles and environmental factors that are detrimental or conducive to sleep.

➤ To allow the patient to apply certain recommendations related to good sleep hygiene, in order to support the effectiveness of other interventions.

Implementation in brief

The patient handout on sleep hygiene can help the patient remember and apply recommendations. It is important to avoid being too rigid when providing these recommendations as they sometimes entail major behavior change (e.g., smoking cessation). An acceptable compromise is often the best solution. As a complement to providing information on sleep hygiene, it is essential to use other behavioral strategies, such as self-monitoring of sleep, limiting time spent in bed, and establishing a time and place for sleep. Scientific studies suggest that intervention on sleep hygiene alone is not sufficient to treat chronic insomnia.

Sleep Hygiene: Maintaining Lifestyle Habits That Promote Good Sleep

The term "sleep hygiene" encompasses a series of recommendations associated with lifestyle habits and environmental factors that are conducive or detrimental to sleep. These factors are rarely the main cause of insomnia, but poor sleep hygiene can worsen the problem. Following is a list of main sleep hygiene recommendations (detailed in the next few pages):

- ✓ Avoid consuming products that contain caffeine 4–6 hours before going to bed.
- ✓ Avoid smoking late in the evening or during nighttime awakenings.
- ✓ Limit alcohol consumption, especially late in the evening.
- ✓ Avoid heavy snacks or foods that stimulate the digestive system late in the evening..
- ✓ Keep the bedroom cool, dark, calm, and comfortable.
- ✓ Physical exercise during the day is excellent but avoid vigorous exercise close to bedtime.

Avoid consuming products that contain caffeine 4–6 hours before going to sleep
■ Caffeine is a central nervous system stimulant.
■ When consumed in the evening, caffeine can delay falling asleep, disturb sleep at night, or make sleep lighter. When taken in large quantities during the day, caffeine can cause withdrawal symptoms in the evening (headaches, palpitations, etc.), thus delaying sleep.
■ Caffeine can be found in coffee, but also in tea, chocolate, certain soft drinks, energy drinks, and a number of over-the-counter medications (e.g., antihistamines for colds and allergies).
■ The greatest concentration of caffeine in the bloodstream is reached 15–45 minutes after consumption, but it takes the body approximately 6 hours to completely eliminate caffeine.

Limit alcohol consumption, especially late in the evening

- Alcohol is a nervous system depressant.
- Some people report that a "nightcap" or small amount of alcohol in the evening can help them fall asleep. This might be true; however, they may also pay a price for this later on: when it is being processed in the body, alcohol can cause agitated and lighter sleep, as well as nighttime or early-morning awakenings.
- Even a moderate quantity of alcohol between dinner and going to bed is likely to disturb sleep.
- Chronic alcohol consumption can disturb sleep, even during periods of sobriety.

Avoid heavy snacks or foods that stimulate the digestive system late in the evening

- Foods that stimulate the digestive system should be avoided, including peanuts, nuts, raw fruits and vegetables, chips, corn, and fatty foods.
- For some individuals, having a light snack and nonalcoholic, noncaffeinated beverage before bedtime appears to facilitate sleep.
- A copious meal late in the evening is detrimental to sleep, given that it will stimulate digestive system activity.
- Snacks should be avoided during nighttime awakenings in order to avoid creating the habit of being awakened by hunger.
- Poor eating habits in general can influence sleep quality and energy level (e.g., an unbalanced diet that is too rich in processed, fatty, sugary, salty, or starchy foods or that lacks certain nutrients, such as proteins or vitamins).

Keep the bedroom cool, dark, calm, and comfortable

- Keep the temperature fairly cool, since warmer temperatures (24 °C or higher) increase awakenings and body movements and diminish both the quality of sleep and the quantity of deep sleep.
- Limit interior and exterior sources of light to avoid interfering with sleep (e.g., using opaque curtains or blinds, or wearing a facemask if necessary).
- Minimize sources of noise (e.g., close the door and windows or use earplugs if limiting sources of noise is not possible): sleep is lighter in a noisy environment, even when one is used to this environment.
- Minimize distractions (e.g., TV and computers) to make the bedroom a place for sleep rather than wakefulness.

Exercise during the day but avoid vigorous exercise in the late evening
■ All regular physical exercise promotes better quality sleep by increasing the quantity of deep sleep. ■ Exercise increases body temperature, which can be followed, for some people, by a cooling-off period that can promote falling asleep (a warm bath roughly 2 hours before going to bed can have the same effect on sleep). ■ Although there are individual differences, for some individuals, engaging in exercise in the middle or late evening can have a stimulating effect and delay sleep onset. ■ The best time to do exercise, in terms of sleep, is the late afternoon or early evening.

Avoid smoking late in the evening and during nighttime awakenings
■ Nicotine is a central nervous system stimulant. ■ Consuming nicotine in the evening or at night can lead to physiological and mental activity that is incompatible with sleep. ■ Nighttime awakenings can be caused by the craving to smoke. ■ Engaging in a process to quit smoking remains the best option.

Clinician guide
Stimulus Control: Recreating a Time and Place for Sleep

Rationale
- To reinforce associations between the sleep period (bedtime, at night), the sleep environment (bed, bedroom), and sleep itself. Good sleepers exhibit strong associations between these factors: a good sleeper can be said to be "conditioned" to sleep in a particular environment (bedroom) and during a particular period (night), which explains why a good sleeper will fall asleep relatively rapidly.
- Over time, insomnia weakens these associations: the bed, bedroom, and sleep period become associated with sleep but also with wakefulness and insomnia (e.g., thinking, worrying, planning, working, watching TV, reading, eating).
- Stimulus control instructions aim at reassociating cues linked to sleep (environment, routine) with sleepiness and aim to eliminate certain behaviors that are incompatible with sleep.

Stimulus control instructions
1. **Set aside at least 1 hour before bedtime for rest and relaxation.**
2. **Go to bed only when you feel sleepy.**
3. **If unable to fall (back) asleep in 15–20 minutes, get out of bed, engage in a calm activity, and go back to bed when sleepiness returns.**
4. **Get up at the same time each morning (using an alarm clock), regardless of how much you slept.**
5. **Reserve the bed and the bedroom exclusively for sleep.**
6. **Limit naps during the day.**

Implementation in brief
Although these instructions seem straightforward, they are challenging for many patients to implement. Importantly, all of the strategies are interdependent: it is crucial for the patient to apply all six strategies, not only those that seem most relevant or require the least effort. If the patient is already applying some of these strategies, it will be easier to focus on those he or she is not yet applying. These strategies may require several weeks of steady application before beneficial effects are experienced. These recommendations apply to people with sleep difficulties, but not necessarily to good sleepers. For

example, watching television in bed before going to sleep is not contra-indicated for someone without insomnia but could be contributing to insomnia of another person. As such, curtailing this behavior might be worth testing.

Take the time to carefully present and discuss the rationale of every strategy with the patient. In subsequent sessions, try to pinpoint barriers or facilitators to implement these recommendations. Specific advice for applying these six strategies is given in the following patient handout. Note that a handout specifically addressing naps and rest periods is available in Chapter 7. Naps are very frequent in persons with brain injury and some individuals may feel they absolutely need them. The need for naps should be carefully evaluated and discussed with patients: timing and duration of naps can be gradually changed, and alternative ways to rest can be explored.

Recreating a Time and Place for Sleep

For good sleepers, the sleep period (nighttime) and sleep environment (the bedroom and bed) are strongly associated with sleep. Insomnia can disrupt these associations over time: the sleep period and environment that should be associated with sleep become associated with wakefulness, becoming tense, worrying about sleep, and eventually insomnia.

Implementing these six essential strategies should help:

1.	Set aside at least 1 hour before bedtime for rest and relaxation.
2.	Go to bed only when you actually feel sleepy
3.	If you are unable to fall (back) asleep in 15–20 minutes, get out of bed, engage in a calm activity, and go back to bed when sleepiness returns.
4.	Get up at the same time each morning (using an alarm clock), regardless of how much you slept, even on weekends.
5.	Reserve the bed and the bedroom exclusively for sleep.
6.	Limit or avoid naps during the day.

 CAUTION:

It is important to apply all six strategies, not only those that seem most relevant to you or require the least effort. These strategies are effective when used together. Just like in a recipe, you cannot expect to have a good result if you're using only some of the ingredients. If you are already applying some of these strategies, focus on the strategies that you are not applying. These strategies may require several weeks of steady application before beneficial effects are experienced. Place this handout well in view to remind yourself of your goals.

---

1. Set aside at least 1 hour before bedtime for rest and relaxation

➤ Later in the evening, avoid sources of mental or emotional activation that can delay your sleep (e.g., working, playing video games, physical exercise, and worrying about the next day).

➤ Choose activities that will facilitate your transition between wakefulness, sleepiness, and sleep (e.g., reading, watching television, or listening to music).

➤ Reserve a specific time in the early evening (and not the late evening) to address worries or problem-solve.

➤ Establish a bedtime routine (e.g., taking a bath, brushing your teeth, removing makeup, or getting into your sleep clothes).

➤ In the late evening, avoid using electronic devices, such as smartphones, tablets, or laptops. The activities you engage in with these devices (e.g., reading your emails, browsing through feeds of social networks, playing video games) can be stimulating, and the light they emit can also be detrimental for sleep.

---

2. Go to bed only when you feel sleepy

➤ Going to bed too early, before you feel sleepy, is likely to delay your sleep and create a stronger association between your bed and bedroom and insomnia.

➤ If you are not sleepy when going to bed, delay your bedtime until you are—you will fall asleep more quickly.

➤ Be attentive to signs of <u>sleepiness</u> (associated with the wakefulness–sleep transition): yawning, heavy eyelids, or itchy or watery eyes.

Sleepiness is not the same thing as fatigue. Sleepiness is associated with sleep drive and is a transitional state between wakefulness and sleep. When feeling sleepy, one may also feel fatigued. However, it is possible to be mentally or physically fatigued without a strong sleep drive, i.e., without being sleepy. Fatigue without sleepiness is often experienced at night by people with insomnia.

---

3. If you are unable to fall (back) asleep in 15–20 minutes, get out of bed, engage in a calm activity, and go back to bed when sleepiness returns

➤ Getting up at night and changing rooms has two advantages: (1) breaking the association between the bed, bedroom, and insomnia and (2) disrupting thought processes that linger when you stay in bed for a long time.

➤ Avoid looking at the time in order to know when you should get out of bed: if you think that 15–20 minutes have gone by or that you will not be able to fall asleep soon (e.g., because you have racing thoughts, you are anxious or agitated), simply get out of bed.

➤ Decide in advance which room you will go to, which activity you will engage in, and what you will need (e.g., in the winter, leave a blanket in the room).

➤ Maintain a relatively dim environment or use a shaded lamp that will not shine directly into your eyes.

➤ Avoid falling asleep in the other room. Go back to bed, but only when you feel sleepy.

➤ Suggested activities: light reading, listening to music, writing, doing crossword puzzles.

➤ Activities to avoid: work or school-related tasks, household tasks, exercise, or using electronic devices.

---

4. Get up at the same time each morning (using an alarm clock), regardless of how much you slept, even on weekends

➤ Use an alarm clock, both during the week and on the weekend, to regulate your sleep cycle and to promote sleep on the following night.

➤ Choose an alarm clock that is loud enough to wake you up, but not too aggressive (e.g., the radio). Put the alarm clock somewhere out of reach so that you need to get up to turn it off.

➤ Plan pleasant, social, or family activities early in the morning in order to increase your motivation to get up.

5. Reserve the bed and the bedroom exclusively for sleep

➤ Avoid the following in your bedroom (during the day and night): reading, watching TV, listening to music or the radio, using a computer or smartphone, eating, working, planning, or worrying. Sexual activities are an exception, since they can lead to a state of relaxation that is conducive to sleep.

➤ Falling asleep to the television or to the radio or other music is especially detrimental: your brain will continue to pay attention to what you are listening to, causing lighter sleep.

➤ As much as possible, it is important to always sleep in the same room and the same bed (avoid sleeping or dozing off in another bed, a couch, or a hammock).

➤ If your room is your living space (e.g., in a hospital, rehabilitation center, or a studio apartment), it is important to set aside a specific space for sleep (the bed) and a space for other activities (other than the bed).

6. Limit or avoid naps during the day

➤ Avoid or limit naps in order to avoid adverse consequences on your sleep the following night. If you feel that you really need a nap, try to follow these recommendations:
  ✓ **Avoid late naps**: the early afternoon is conducive to falling asleep quickly, but a late-afternoon or evening nap can disturb sleep of the following night.
  ✓ **Keep the nap brief**: 15–30 minutes naps are more effective than longer naps. Short naps are sufficient to reduce sleepiness, while long naps are usually followed by a prolonged transition period before feeling fully alert (e.g., feeling groggy).
  ✓ **Nap in your bed**: naps should be taken in the same place as sleep at night, i.e., in your bed.

➤ Try to find alternatives to naps in order to deal with sleepiness or fatigue during the day: listen to music, take a walk outside, exercise (e.g., yoga, swimming), take a bath, or engage in a pleasant or social activity. You may find that these activities replenish your energy levels and provide other benefits that you may miss out on if sleeping.

Clinician guide
Restriction of Time in Bed: Limiting the Time Spent in Bed to Actual Sleeping Time

Rationale

> One of the most common strategies for dealing with insomnia is spending more time in bed to increase opportunities for sleep or rest (e.g., going to bed earlier, getting up later, and taking naps). In the long term, this can contribute to perpetuate sleep difficulties.

> Restriction of time in bed, also called "sleep restriction" or "bedtime restriction," is an effective behavioral strategy which consists in limiting the number of hours spent in bed as close as possible to the number of hours of actual sleep through a "sleep window". The main objective is to improve sleep efficiency and quality, but not necessarily to increase the amount of sleep. This can be achieved once sleep efficiency is optimized, i.e., after a few weeks of application.

> Initially, reducing the amount of time spent in bed will also reduce the amount of sleep, thus creating mild sleep deprivation. After a few nights, this slight sleep deprivation will increase homeostatic sleep drive and may help to reduce time to sleep onset and sleep fragmentation.

> Sleep duration will come closer to the (newly reduced) amount of time spent in bed.

> In time, sleep will become more consolidated. This will promote deeper sleep, decrease time spent awake, and thereby improve sleep efficiency.

> By maintaining a set bedtime and rising time, this will also regulate the biological clock in order to allow sleep to come when needed.

> Once sleep efficiency is improved, time spent in bed can be <u>very</u> gradually increased (by 15–20 minutes each week) until an optimal sleep window is found.

Implementation in brief

Spending less time in bed in order to sleep better can seem counterintuitive. Many patients will at first be surprised or skeptical. It is, therefore, crucial to thoroughly explain the rationale behind this strategy. **To ensure the strategy's effectiveness, the time spent in bed must be limited consistently for several weeks (generally 3–4) in order to**

achieve established goals. Although response time varies from one individual to another, it is not unusual for 2 to 3 weeks of rigorous application to be needed before beneficial effects even begin to be experienced. The clinician's role is, therefore, to keep the patient motivated, to normalize his or her experience, and to encourage continued application of the strategy. A certain level of flexibility is warranted if the clinician is unsure about patient adherence to the sleep window: deciding on a sleep window should ideally be done collaboratively with the patient, taking into account the latter's willingness and perception of being able to adhere to the sleep window. While a too large sleep window can produce less rapid or optimal outcomes, an approach that is too rigid or prescriptive can lead to poor adherence.

Four steps will be necessary:

STEP 1. Work together with the patient in determining his or her first sleep window

- ➤ The patient's **sleep window** is the period when sleep is permitted, and outside of which sleep should be avoided. The window is defined by a set bedtime and rising time.
- ➤ The duration of the sleep window is periodically reviewed (generally each week) and adjusted as necessary.
- ➤ The duration of the first sleep window is equal to the number or hours slept on average each night over the past week or two (an additional 30 minutes can be added for more flexibility or adherence). If possible, this number of hours should be calculated based on the sleep diary. Otherwise, it can be approximated by asking the patient about his or her sleep habits.
- ➤ The sleep window must be applied every day, whether during the week or on the weekend, regardless of sleep quantity or quality.
- ➤ The sleep window is generally maintained for 1 week, after which it is adjusted on a weekly basis according to sleep efficiency.

  Important safety concern

In order to avoid excessive sleepiness during the day, the duration of the sleep window (time spent in bed) should not be reduced to less than 5 hours per night. This is especially important with people engaging in activities where sleepiness can be hazardous (e.g., driving long distances, manipulating potentially harmful machinery or equipment).

STEP 2. Determine bedtime and rising time together with the patient

- ➤ Determine a set bedtime and rising time that will define the sleep window, while taking into account the patient's work, obligations, and lifestyle. The patient should actively participate in choosing his or her schedule. For example, one might prefer staying up later and getting up later or the reverse.
- ➤ The patient should try to stay awake until the established bedtime and get up at the established time, even if he or she is still sleeping.
- ➤ The set sleep window will remain unchanged for at least 1 week.
- ➤ For the first sleep window, it is generally recommended to choose a rising time that can be maintained for several weeks and a corresponding bedtime that can gradually be moved earlier over the weeks. It is easier to gradually add sleep time in the evening as opposed to later in the morning.
- ➤ Stress the importance of using an alarm clock or alarm function for rising, or ask someone living with the patient to wake him or her up in order to respect the established rising time and hence ensure the strategy's effectiveness.

STEP 3. Encourage the patient to apply the sleep window diligently during the week

- ➤ Anticipate challenges and consult the list of "Common obstacles and solutions while implementing restriction of time in bed" mentioned later to prepare the patient for the upcoming week.
- ➤ Encourage the patient to adopt a scientific attitude and test out if the strategy works at least until the next session.

STEP 4. Adjust the sleep window together with the patient on a weekly basis

- ➤ Each week during the implementation of restriction of time in bed, it is very important to evaluate sleep efficiency as calculated from the sleep diary (the percentage of time spent in bed during which the patient is actually sleeping). The sleep window will be adjusted according to sleep efficiency while taking into consideration the patient's condition (e.g., presence of sleepiness or difficulty with respecting the sleep window).
- ➤ Here is how to adjust the sleep window according to sleep efficiency:
  - ⇨ $\geq 85\%$: extend the window by 15–20 minutes for the following week, by moving bedtime earlier or pushing rising time later.
  - ⇨ $< 80\%$: reduce the window by 15–20 minutes for the following week, by pushing bedtime later or moving rising time earlier.
  - ⇨ 80–85%: maintain the same window for the following week.

➤ These criteria can be made more flexible in order to extend the window (e.g., sleep efficiency ≥ 80% or even less) in cases where:
  ⇨ The patient exhibited very low sleep efficiency at the beginning of the intervention (e.g., <60%).
  ⇨ Daytime sleepiness is very strong and incapacitating.
  ⇨ The patient is significantly struggling to respect the sleep window or is very anxious about applying this strategy. For individuals who are very concerned about a lack of sleep or about the application of this strategy, it can be possible to make more frequent adjustments to the sleep window (e.g., by phone between sessions).

Common obstacles and solutions while implementing restriction of time in bed

The patient reports feeling sleepy during the day

➤ Normalize the sleepiness: during the first few weeks, sleep duration may be slightly reduced, causing sleepiness during the day.
➤ **This side effect is normal and temporary**, it is actually a good sign that the strategy is working (i.e., sleep drive is increased).
➤ Point out the positive side: the patient might wonder if he or she will be able to stay awake until bedtime, which can help lower performance anxiety. Instead of being worried about not sleeping that night, he or she will be impatient to go to bed.

 CAUTION:

Again, in applying this procedure, caution is recommended if the patient holds a job or practices a leisure activity in which sleepiness can be a hazard (e.g., driving a car or handling machinery).

The patient reports feeling sleepy in the evening and has difficulty pushing back bedtime

➤ Plan activities to avoid dozing off in the evening.
➤ Avoid long, passive activities (e.g., watching TV for 3 hours in a row).
➤ Prioritize pleasant activities and alternate between activities.
➤ Draw up a list of potential activities together with the patient and suggest that he or she try them out to determine which ones are effective against sleepiness.
➤ Seek the collaboration of a family member living with the patient to help him or her avoiding dozing off too early.

The patient reports having difficulty getting up at the same time each morning

➢ Encourage patients to always use an alarm clock, even if they feel they do not need it.

➢ Encourage the patient to plan (social and pleasant) activities early in the morning to increase motivation to get up.

➢ Encourage the patient to associate getting up with activities rather than only with the strategy of restricting time spent in bed.

➢ Help the patient develop a morning routine that suits him or her.

The patient worries about the consequences of restriction of time in bed on the next day

➢ If the patient is worried about being unable to function the next day, he or she can be reminded that:

  • The duration of the first sleep window is about equal to the average number of hours he or she has slept over the past week.

  • As soon as sleep efficiency improves, the window will be extended.

  • The only direct consequence of the strategy is sleepiness, which is temporary and gradually goes away after a few weeks.

  • Sleepiness will increase sleep drive and thus potentially help the body and brain to fall asleep more easily and stay asleep for a longer period of time.

  • Fatigue may increase slightly but there should not be any significant consequence (but remain alert whether sleepiness is an issue if the person needs to drive or operate machinery).

Limiting the Time Spent in Bed to Actual Sleeping Time

One of the strategies that people commonly use to cope with insomnia is to spend more time in bed in hope of getting more rest: going to bed earlier, getting up later, or taking naps. These practices can feel beneficial in the short term, but they can be detrimental in the long term: spending too much time awake in bed tends to fragment sleep and diminish the association between the bedroom and sleep and therefore perpetuate insomnia.

One strategy that has received much evidence in research is to limit the time spent in bed to actual sleeping time.

- This strategy is very effective for decreasing sleep fragmentation and increasing sleep quality.
- The initial effect is to produce a mild state of sleep deprivation, which makes it easier to fall asleep and improves the continuity of sleep through the night.
- In the beginning, the goal is to improve sleep quality and efficiency, but not necessarily to increase your total sleep time. In the longer term, the duration of your sleep may increase, once the quality of your sleep has improved.

This figure illustrates how spending more or less time in bed can influence sleep quality.

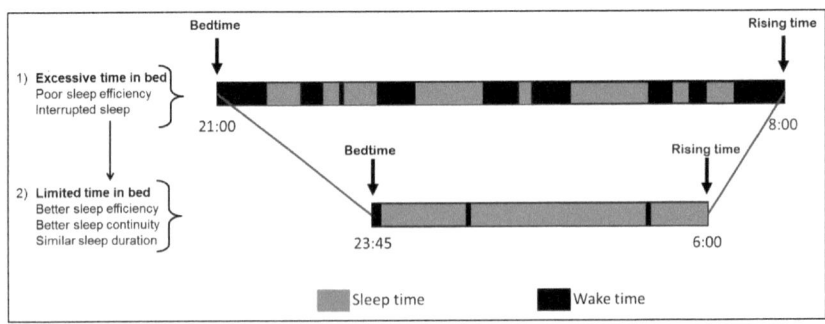

To apply this strategy, you can follow these steps:

1.	Determine the duration of your sleep window based on the amount of time you actually sleep
2.	Choose a set bedtime and rising time to define the sleep window
3.	Apply the sleep window each night for 1 week
4.	Each week, adjust the sleep window based on your sleep efficiency and how sleepy you are during the day

1. Determine the duration of your sleep window based on the amount of time you actually sleep

The **sleep window** is a period of time in which sleep is permitted, and outside of which sleep should be avoided. The sleep window is defined by a set bedtime and rising time, **and it must be followed each night, whether during the week or on the weekend.**

The duration of the first sleep window is equal to the average number of hours you have slept each night over the past week or 2 weeks + 30 minutes. Your therapist can help you estimate this duration based on your habits or using your sleep diary. Here is an example:

Day	Mon Oct 21	Tues Oct 22	Wed Oct 23	Thu Oct 24	Fri Oct 25	Sat Oct 26	Sun Oct 27
Hours of sleep	7 h	6 h	5 h 30	6 h	6 h 15	5 h 45	5 h 30

Average sleep time = (Total hours of sleep ÷ Number of days) = (42 hours total ÷ 7 days) = 6 hours, to which is added 30 minutes

➢ **The duration of the first sleep window will be 6.5 hours**

 CAUTION:

To avoid significant sleepiness during the day, **the sleep window should never be less than 5 hours in duration**, even if you generally sleep less than this amount.

2. Choose a set bedtime and rising time to define the sleep window

➢ These times will be set for at least 1 week.
➢ For example, for a 6-hour sleep window, possible bedtimes and rising times might include:
  ✓ 11:30 p.m. to 5:30 a.m.
  ✓ 12 a.m. to 6 a.m.
  ✓ 12:30 a.m. to 6:30 a.m.
➢ Choose bedtime and rising times that fit well with your life and activities and your preferences.
➢ Explore strategies to try to apply the sleep window as diligently as possible.

3. Apply the sleep window each night for 1 week. You will subsequently readjust this window based on your sleep efficiency for the week.

What to expect

➢ The side effect of this strategy of restricting time spent in bed is that you will feel sleepier during the day. This is normal and temporary. After 1 or 2 weeks, you will realize that, in spite of spending less time in bed, you are functioning just as well during the day. Exercise caution if you need to drive or use hazardous machinery.

4. Each week, adjust the sleep window based on your sleep efficiency and how sleepy you are during the day

➢ If your sleep efficiency improves (or if you are very sleepy), you may increase your sleep window by 15–20 minutes.
➢ Continue to adjust your sleep window each week until you achieve a satisfactory duration of sleep combined with good sleep efficiency (85%). You may need to apply this strategy for several weeks before achieving this result.

How to adjust your sleep window:

$$\text{Sleep efficiency} = \frac{\text{Total sleep time (in minutes)}}{\text{Time spent in bed at night (in minutes)}} \times 100$$

If your sleep efficiency is **above 85%** OR If you are very sleepy during the day (much sleepier than before you began using this strategy). ►	**Increase your sleep window** by 15–20 minutes for the following week. You may decide to go to bed earlier at night or get out of bed later in the morning.
If your sleep efficiency is **below 80%** AND You are not too sleepy during the day. ►	**Reduce your sleep window** by 15–20 minutes for the following week. You may go to bed later at night or get out of bed earlier in the morning. The essential point is to reduce the amount of time that you spend in bed.If you have been unable to apply the sleep window in the past week, you may also try maintaining the same bedtime and rising time for one more week.
If your sleep efficiency is **between 80 and 85%.** ►	**Maintain the same sleep window** for another week.

Clinician guide
Brief Cognitive Therapy: Promoting Beliefs and Attitudes That are Conducive to Sleep

Rationale
- ➤ To clarify certain sleep-related facts and foster realistic expectations.
- ➤ To help the patient avoid dramatizing the consequences of insomnia out of proportion and to consider other explanations for issues experienced during the day.
- ➤ To help the patient become aware of the negative sleep-related consequences of excessive thinking and worrying about sleep.
- ➤ To suggest strategies for managing worries in the evening or at night.

Implementation in brief
- ➤ Administer the **Dysfunctional Beliefs and Attitudes about Sleep** questionnaire (available in Chapter 8) in order to identify and focus the discussion on statements that the patient endorses more strongly.
- ➤ Provide the patient handout on beliefs and attitudes about sleep and discuss each topic with the patient: What is his or her opinion? Does he or she agree with what is suggested? In the patient's view, how can his or her attitudes or beliefs interact with sleep or the consequences of insomnia? With some brain injured individuals, you may engage in Socratic questioning and other cognitive therapy techniques if appropriate.
- ➤ As a complement, present the handout "Strategies for better management of worries when going to bed or during nighttime awakenings" and teach relaxation and breathing techniques.

 **My Motivating Activities**

If you feel sleepy in the evening but need to wait until your appropriate bedtime:

- Plan activities to avoid dozing off in the evening
- Avoid long, passive activities (e.g., watching TV for 2 hours in a row)
- Plan pleasant activities and alternate between activities
- Collect a list of potential activities and try them out to determine which ones are effective against sleepiness

My motivating activities for the evening:

_____

_____

_____

_____

_____

What to do if you find it difficult to get up at the same time each morning:

- Plan social and pleasant activities early in the morning to increase motivation to get up;
- Try thinking of getting up early as more time to do your favorite activities;
- Develop a morning routine you enjoy.

My motivating activities for the morning:

_____

_____

_____

_____

_____

 Beliefs and Attitudes That Promote Good Sleep

Your beliefs and attitudes about sleep can actually contribute to your insomnia. By changing your perception and understanding of a problem (such as insomnia), you can reduce your emotional distress, which can be beneficial for your sleep.

The goal here is not to deny or minimize your sleep difficulties or their effect on your daily functioning. We know these are very real and very common after a brain injury. Rather, the goal is to encourage you to consider the possibility that some of your beliefs may not be helpful and that exploring different ways of thinking about sleep and insomnia can be beneficial.

Following is a list of helpful attitudes:

Review the causes of insomnia
Maintain realistic expectations toward sleep
Do not try to force sleep
Avoid giving sleep too much importance
Avoid blowing the consequences of sleep difficulties out of proportion
Develop a tolerance for variations in your sleep
Avoid comparing your sleep to before your accident

The boxes below explain why these attitudes are helpful:

Review the causes of insomnia

➢ Looking for one absolute cause behind sleep difficulties gives the individual little or no control over these difficulties. There are always several causes to insomnia.

➢ Although it is important to acknowledge that certain unchangeable factors can contribute to insomnia, feeling a lack of control over insomnia can lead to a sense of despair and powerlessness.

➢ Regardless of the factors that have led to the onset of insomnia, certain behaviors and attitudes that are adopted over time can be changed, such as sleep–wake schedules, habits, and beliefs and attitudes toward sleep.

Maintain realistic expectations toward sleep

➤ It is often said that 8 hours of sleep are needed for everyone each night in order to feel refreshed. This is a myth: the amount of sleep needed varies substantially from one person to another. Some function very well on less than this average amount, while others will need more to feel well rested.

➤ Significant individual differences can also be observed in terms of how quickly individuals fall asleep, the number of nighttime awakenings they experience, and the general quality of their sleep. For example, it may sometimes be frustrating to see a spouse fall asleep very easily while you are struggling. Remember that just like personality, height, or preference, everyone is different.

➤ It is best to avoid pressuring yourself to achieve certain standards: putting pressure on yourself disturbs rather than facilitates sleep.

➤ It is also preferable not to compare your sleep with that of others, since this can lead to frustration or disappointment.

Do not try to force sleep

➤ It is possible to control certain circumstances, thoughts, and habits that promote good sleep, but not to control sleep itself: sleep cannot be induced on command, it is dependent on complex brain and body systems.

➤ Trying too hard and giving too much importance to falling asleep will produce anxiety or worrying therefore delaying sleep.

➤ Many people who suffer from insomnia are prone to falling asleep in unexpected situations, when not trying to sleep, for example, while watching TV or reading, because they do not pressure themselves in these contexts.

➤ Following the recommendations in this intervention including respecting your sleep window will gradually help relieve the pressure you put on yourself and let your brain and body readjust to produce sleep more regularly.

Avoid giving sleep too much importance

➢ Some people plan their social, work, and family activities based on the quantity and quality of their sleep over the previous night. This behavior tends to reinforce the sense of being a victim while creating anxiety and pressure to sleep well the following night.

Avoid blowing the consequences of sleep difficulties out of proportion

➢ It is true that a poor night of sleep can disturb personal functioning the next day (by leading to fatigue, irritability, and discouragement). However, in general, the consequences are fairly minor and do not prevent the completion of everyday activities. Furthermore, a poor night (or a few poor nights) is often followed by a better night of recovery.

➢ Moreover, a poor night of sleep will not necessarily be followed by a bad day, just as a good night of sleep will not necessarily be followed by a good day.

➢ This means that sleep is not the only factor explaining our state the next day: other factors, such as stress, health, motivation, and our choice of activities, are probably as important.

➢ Anticipating and fearing the consequences of a poor night of sleep only worsen the situation and create worrying that is detrimental to sleep. If you notice yourself worrying about your sleep during the day, notice and accept that these thoughts are going through your mind, but do not give them particular attention: refocus on your activity in the present moment.

Develop a tolerance for variations in your sleep

➢ It is normal for sleep quality or quantity to vary. Even persons without insomnia or TBI have nights that are not as refreshing as others.

➢ After a poor night of sleep, it is important to continue to follow a regular routine and honor commitments, thus helping to get your mind off of insomnia and its consequences.

➢ Planning pleasant activities after a poor night of sleep helps you realize that insomnia does not prevent you from doing what you want.

➢ If possible, adapt your schedule. For example, you could alternate between different types of tasks, plan refreshing breaks, or place demanding tasks at a time when you know you will have more energy.

Avoid comparing your sleep to before your accident

➤ Did you sleep perfectly well every single night before your accident? When dealing with a new illness or condition, many people will have a "good old days" bias and forget that they quite often felt fatigue, irritability, forgetfulness, lack of concentration, or headaches even when they did not have the illness or condition.

➤ Instead, try to think about what would be an adequate night of sleep most of the time or an acceptable energy level given your current circumstances.

➤ Instead of looking back, look forward at the progress you make every day.

Strategies for Better Management of Worries When Going to Bed or During Nighttime Awakenings

After a TBI, it is not unusual to simultaneously experience multiple stressful events. Concerns about your future and your health (including your sleep and energy level) can arise. Excessive worrying in the evening or at night can be contributing to your sleep difficulties. Here are a few that help you to deal with your worries more effectively:

➤ **Avoid giving your worries or thoughts too much importance.**
   We all have thoughts and worries, especially when we have real problems to deal with. When worrying takes up too much energy and interferes with sleep, however, it can be useful to take a step back and notice what is happening in our mind. We tend to engage with our worries, feeling that if we stop worrying, we might lose control over the situation. Worries are just thoughts, they are not an effective way to solve problems. Instead of engaging with your worries, take a moment to notice: "I am worrying right now." You can then try letting these thoughts go by without engaging with them, without giving too much importance or attention. Accept that you have these thoughts, but instead of focusing on them, choose instead to focus on something else, for example, your breathing.

➤ **Plan specific times to address your worries.**
   Rather than allowing worries to take over your mind at any time of day or night, try to plan a specific time and place during the day (e.g., from 7:00 to 7:15 PM in a chair that you do not use very often) when you can be free to address them. If worries arise at other times, acknowledge that you have these worries and note them down and remind yourself that you will give them your full attention at the established time and place.

➤ **Plan specific times for problem-solving.**
   If you want to solve problems, then plan this activity as you would any other. Do not engage in problem-solving too close to bedtime or when in bed, rather plan a specific time in the day or early evening to do so. Use a notebook, planner, or smartphone to note down your worries, reminders, or problems to solve. Once you have these in writing, you will know you can give them more attention at a better time.

> ## What is effective problem-solving?

Try the following steps to effectively problem-solve. This can take time, ask for help, and advice and give yourself a chance to try several solutions.

Steps to problem-solve effectively
Write down what the problem in *specific* terms
_____
Imagine various solutions to the problems (even those which seem far-fetched)
_____ _____ _____ _____
_____ _____ _____ _____
Write down and weigh the pros and cons of each solution
Solution 1   Pros: Cons:
Solution 2   Pros: Cons:
Solution 3   Pros: Cons:
4. Figure out what is the best solution (often there is no perfect solution)
_____
5. Try out the solution, give it a good chance, and evaluate the results
_____
6. If the result is satisfactory, great, if not, go to your next best solution or start the process again
_____

> **Use breathing or relaxation strategies.**

To quiet down your mind when going to bed, try breathing, relaxation, or visualization strategies. Following are some very simple yet quite effective breathing techniques. Regular practice of these will make them easier to apply.

Paying attention to your breathing

Direct your attention to your breathing and try to slow it down. Concentrate on the sensation of air entering and leaving your nostrils. Notice that the air is cool when entering your body and warmer when exhaling. You may also notice sensations in you abdomen or chest when you breathe in or out. You may also simply focus your attention on the sounds of your breathing. If your mind wanders and worries arise, just try to accept these thoughts without blocking them, and turn your attention back to your breathing.

Abdominal breathing

Put one hand on your chest and the other on your abdomen. Without forcing it, try to breathe by filling your abdomen rather than chest. You should feel your abdomen expand as you breathe in. The hand on your chest should hardly move. With practice, you will be able to spontaneously breathe more from the abdomen, which is more strongly associated with relaxation than chest breathing.

Extending your breath

Breathe in through your nose and **slowly** exhale through your mouth or nose. Without forcing in any way, extend your breath so that you slow down your inhalation and exhalation. If you feel comfortable, you can even take pauses of 1 to 2 seconds between your inhalations and exhalations.

Clinician guide
Motivational Strategies When Encountering Resistance

When encountering resistance with a patient, it may be helpful to suspend the intervention temporarily and engage in a motivational approach: it is important to express empathy and recognize the challenges of the intervention. Take a step back from the more directive approach and roll with resistance, while reinforcing the patient's self-efficacy. This may even require a few sessions. The following questions can guide your approach.

Sample questions to foster change
- What would you like to change about your sleep or fatigue? - What concerns you about your present situation with you sleep–wake cycle? - How would you like things to be different? - Why is this important to you? How much do you want to change? - What would be the advantages of making a change or putting efforts in this intervention? - How confident do you feel about your ability to implement the strategies we have talked about? - On a scale of 0–10 where 0 is not at all confident, and 10 is absolutely confident, how would you rate yourself? (Discuss the result. For example: Why did you say 6 rather than 2 or 3)? - What makes you believe that you could succeed if you decide to make a change? - Have you made changes in your life or habits before? How did you manage to change? Which of your personal strengths helped you succeed in the past? - Who could you use these strengths during this intervention? - What would you be willing to try first? - How confident do you feel you can do this? (use confidence scale 0–10 as needed)

Adapted from Arechiga A. (2010). Facilitating Health Behavior Change. In D. Wedding & M.L. Stuber (Eds), Behavior and Medicine, 5th ed., Cambridge, MA Toronto: Hogrefe & Huber Publishers, p. 148.

Clinician guide
Clinical Challenges and Solutions to Adapt CBT for Insomnia to the Context of TBI

Cognitive deficits
- Build in repetition to ensure encoding of rationale of treatment strategies and nature of recommendations.
- Closely monitor the efficacy of self-monitoring (e.g., sleep diary) to ensure comprehension and effective use. Use shorter, simplified versions of self-monitoring tools (e.g., sleep diaries) and other instruments as necessary.
- Prefer shorter sessions (e.g., 20–30 min instead of 50–60 min) to avoid fatigue and adjust the timing/rhythm of session to the patient.
- Schedule CBT sessions at a time when the energy level is optimal.
- Prioritize behavioral strategies and introduce them gradually (e.g., restriction of time in bed alone initially, then gradually implement stimulus control).
- If necessary, simplify or avoid more complex or introspective strategies, such as cognitive restructuring (e.g., use the Dysfunctional Beliefs and Attitudes about Sleep scale to explore cognitions and offer alternative interpretations, attitudes).
- Provide simplified written and visual summaries of each CBT strategy. Use metaphors, pictograms, or cue cards to help encoding and retention of treatment material.
- Use portable electronic devices (e.g., smartphones) to foster compliance (e.g., set reminders to complete sleep diaries or to apply sleep window, refer to one of many available sleep apps).
- Consider the involvement of a significant other to whom the rationale and application of each strategy are described to promote compliance and support.

Physical limitations
- Evaluate how physical conditions, pain, mobility issues, and motor impairments can interfere with the implementation of CBT strategies. Contact and stay in touch with treating physician or other health-care professionals about physical health particularities and medication use.
- Discuss with the patient his/her perceptions and beliefs about the interrelationships between sleep, pain, fatigue, and physical functioning.
- For patients with limited mobility, consider a modified version of stimulus control instructions (e.g., sitting up in bed when unable to fall asleep instead of getting out of bed and going to another room).
- When inactivity or physical deconditioning is an issue, gradually reintegrate simple, varied, and adapted activities.

Behavioral particularities
- Ensure that the patient has sufficient self-awareness and motivation before starting the intervention.
- Provide structured, targeted session agendas to avoid distractions.
- Immediately address disinhibition or inappropriate behavior to reiterate the purpose of the sessions.
- Provide reinforcement and encouragement throughout the treatment process, especially with patients with apathy or lack of initiative.
- Remain flexible (e.g., to missed appointments, lack of compliance) and involve patients in problem-solving.
- As alcohol and recreational drug use is common, provide information on their impact on sleep and fatigue, and monitor their use during treatment.
- For patients with significant initiation or motivational issues, consider motivational interviewing techniques to build self-efficacy.

Anxiety and depression symptoms
- Carefully assess the presence of anxiety and depression symptoms, discuss them with patients, and inform patients on their interaction with sleep—wake difficulties.
- Promote balance between activities (e.g., behavioral activation techniques to encourage pleasant, rewarding, useful, social, and physical activities).
- Be flexible when implementing behavioral strategies when significant anxiety symptoms are present (e.g., gradually decreasing time spent in bed rather than drastically decreasing it initially and then gradually increasing it).
- Encourage patients to seek support from their family and friends.

Intervention Tools for Post-TBI Fatigue

OVERVIEW

This chapter is a compendium of intervention tools for post-TBI fatigue. These tools should be used with a thorough understanding of their evidence base, rationale, and procedures, and after an exhaustive evaluation. It is, therefore, important to refer to Chapters 1 to 5 to ensure adequate preparation for intervention. This chapter includes the following Clinician Guides and corresponding handouts for patients:

Insomnia and Fatigue after Traumatic Brain Injury
DOI: https://doi.org/10.1016/B978-0-12-811316-5.00007-0

Clinician Guides	Patient Handouts
• Overview of intervention strategies for post-TBI fatigue	• Self-management of energy and fatigue • Helping a family member or friend manage fatigue (for significant others)
• Establishing effective self-monitoring with the energy/activity diary	• An essential tool: the energy/activity diary
• Presenting basic facts about fatigue and understanding the vicious circle of fatigue and the benefits of better energy management	• Fatigue following a traumatic brain injury • The vicious circle of fatigue • The positive cycle of effective energy management
• Understanding the connection between lifestyle habits and fatigue	• Healthy habits to optimize energy
• Improving self-perception of signs of fatigue	• Recognizing the signs of fatigue
• Understanding energy level fluctuations and the activity—fatigue connection	• Understanding the activity—fatigue connection (example) • Identifying sources of energy and fatigue
• Counteracting inactivity by gradually increasing activity level and planning rest periods	• Different ways to rest • Recommendations concerning naps and rest periods
• Strategies to adapt activities in order to manage energy levels effectively	• Adapting activities to minimize fatigue • Identifying high-risk situations
• Promoting attitudes and expectations for good energy management	• Maintaining a balance between different types of activities • Reintegrating avoided activities and integrating new activities • Maintaining realistic expectations about my energy levels
• Gradually increasing physical activity to better manage fatigue	• Increasing physical activity to fight fatigue

Clinician guide
Overview of Intervention Strategies for Post-TBI Fatigue

	Intervention	Goals
PSYCHOEDUCATION	**Establishing self-monitoring with the energy/activity diary**	• To document fatigue level; • To analyze the connection between activities and energy or fatigue level; • To apply behavioral strategies; • To keep track of progress.
	Understanding the vicious circle of fatigue and the benefits of better energy management	• To identify behaviors that contribute to perpetuating fatigue; • To raise awareness of the importance of better managing activity levels for better energy management.
	Understanding the connection between lifestyle habits and fatigue	• To identify lifestyle habits that may be contributing to fatigue.
COGNITIVE-BEHAVIORAL INTERVENTIONS	**Improving self-perception of signs of fatigue**	• To identify one's signs of fatigue; • To better identify and respect one's limits.
	Understanding energy level fluctuations and the activity–fatigue connection	• To understand energy level fluctuations as they relate to activities.
	Counteracting inactivity by gradually increasing activity level and planning rest periods	• To gradually reduce inactive time and increase active time; • To plan both activity and rest periods.
	Strategies to adapt activities in order to manage energy levels effectively	• To learn to manage energy before, during, and after activities; • To avoid the overexertion–inactivity cycle.

| COGNITIVE-BEHAVIORAL INTERVENTIONS | Promoting attitudes and expectations for good energy management | • To promote realistic expectations with regard to current personal functioning;
• To maintain balance between different types of activities;
• To reintegrate certain activities. |
| | Gradually increasing physical activity | • To gradually incorporate physical activity into the routine;
• To work toward realistic and lasting changes. |

NOTE: Chapter 8 presents an eight-session protocol which was evaluated in a clinical case series integrating intervention for both insomnia and fatigue (Ouellet & Morin, 2007, Archives of Physical Medicine and Rehabilitation, 88(12):1581−1592).

 Self-Management of Energy

During this intervention, you will develop skills to better manage your fatigue and energy levels. This intervention is unlikely to eliminate completely your fatigue, but you will learn to manage your energy and activities more effectively so that you can increase your quality of life and engage in the important activities in your life with satisfaction. Here are a few key ingredients for success with this approach:

➤ **Commit and keep an open mind**
  In the next few weeks, try to understand the links between your energy or fatigue levels and the different types of activities you engage in. Make energy management a priority so that you can test out different strategies.

➤ **Take your time and expect changes to take time**
  Do not expect results within a week or two. Learning new habits takes time. The pace of your improvement will vary depending on the nature and severity of your fatigue problem, the presence of other physical or psychological problems, and your motivation.

➤ **Make sure your loved ones are on board**
  All through the intervention, discuss why and how you are changing your activities with your loved ones so that they can understand your goals, encourage, and help you. During this period, this may mean some readjustments in roles for you and for your loved ones: for example, since your accident you may have abandoned or reduced certain activities, or you may need more help from family members or friends for certain tasks. Effective energy management will mean trying to gradually reintegrate certain activities or tasks or trying new activities. You can explain to your loved ones that being supportive can at times mean providing some help, but at other times it can mean providing less help, and letting you test out what you are able to accomplish while respecting your limits.

➤ **Be tolerant toward yourself and stay realistic**
  When it comes to managing energy, many of us often have unrealistic expectations: we want to achieve too much given the time, resources, or energy at hand. This can be quite frustrating and

disappointing. In this intervention, you will learn to set achievable goals and to be positive about what you have accomplished rather than focusing on what you have not done.

➤ **Avoid constantly comparing yourself to "before the accident"**
"Before the accident I could have done this without being tired" This type of thinking can be very frustrating. It can make you feel helpless and you may give up even trying to get back to certain activities. Remember that it is easy to idealize how things were before. "Despite my fatigue, this is what I have accomplished today" will be a more encouraging way to look at things. In this intervention, we will invite you to focus on small steps to gradually resume certain activities or try new ones: the goal is to feel satisfied with completing shorter periods of an activity, or part of an activity, with an acceptable level of energy or fatigue, given your current circumstances. Gradually, you will be able to feel more confident and build up more stamina when engaging in your activities. Shift your focus toward the present and on your recent progress, this will be much more encouraging for you.

➤ **Give yourself a chance and maintain a scientific attitude**
Before concluding that the intervention does not work for you, be sure to test out the recommendations thoroughly for several weeks and see what happens. Keep an open mind, observe yourself, you will at least learn more about your habits and ways of functioning which should be helpful.

 Helping a Family Member or Friend Manage Fatigue

Fatigue is an extremely common and significant problem for persons who have had a traumatic brain injury. Your family member or friend is in the process of trying to developing personal management skills to better manage their energy levels: this will imply recognizing signs of fatigue, adapting activities, increasing certain activities (e.g., exercise), and having a more positive focus on what can be done relative to the energy available. This intervention will not likely completely eliminate fatigue. The goal of intervention is rather for your loved one to learn to manage energy more effectively in order to maintain a good quality of life and feel satisfied when engaging in different activities.

What you can do to help your family member or friend?

➤ Be encouraging. Taking charge of fatigue problems requires effort and discipline. Encourage your family member or friend to apply the suggested strategies and remind him or her that several weeks might be needed before noticeable improvement occurs.

➤ Avoid seeing your family member or friend's fatigue as laziness or a lack of willpower. Fatigue is a very real problem following a traumatic brain injury. It is very common and can be quite incapacitating. For example, fatigue can have a major impact on one's capacity to return to work.

➤ Encourage your family member or friend to engage in regular physical exercise (but not too close to bedtime), which helps improve energy level, sleep, and mood. You may even improve your own health by accompanying your loved one in physical activities.

➤ Encourage him or her to stay active, while respecting his or her personal rhythms and capacity.

➤ If you notice that your loved one is overdoing an activity, be positive about what has already been accomplished, suggest a break, or suggest alternating with another activity. The initial activity may be continued at a later time. You can use the battery analogy: *"Remember not use up all your energy, it will take less time for your battery to recharge if it is not completely empty."*

➤ Naps and rest periods are not the only solutions to fatigue. You might also suggest alternative activities that can renew energy or just refresh the mind, such as social, enjoyable, or fulfilling activities: some examples are taking a walk, listening to music, calling a friend.

➤ As much as possible, avoid indefinitely handling tasks that seem too exhausting for your family member or friend. By letting him or her reengage in these activities, you will help him or her to gradually learn to resume these tasks with better energy management.

➤ Avoid jumping to the conclusion that your friend or family member's behavior is only due to fatigue when he or she is irritable, exhibiting organization problems, struggling with his or her concentration or memory, or being aggressive. Other factors might also be involved.

➤ Help establish a regular sleep—wake schedule, healthy eating habits, and regular meal times.

Clinician guide
Establishing Effective Self-Monitoring With the Energy/Activity Diary

Rationale and benefits of using an energy/activity diary

Restores the patient's sense of control over his or her energy and activities	➤ By enabling observation of energy level variations, signs of fatigue, and their connection with activities that were done; ➤ By identifying global patterns of behavior linked to energy levels; ➤ By revealing connections with the progression of fatigue over a given activity, day, or week; ➤ By creating emotional distance from fatigue problems; ➤ By allowing the patient to consider changes to better manage his or her energy.
Gives the patient an active role in managing his or her energy	➤ By allowing the patient to begin to structure his or her own time; ➤ By allowing observation of the patient's activity schedule and energy level fluctuations; ➤ By suggesting solutions for improving energy level; ➤ By helping to establish behaviors that enable self-management of energy.
Documents fatigue	➤ By specifying the intensity of fatigue at different times of the day; ➤ By revealing that some activities can be done in spite of fatigue and avoid catastrophizing; ➤ By promoting a better understanding of fatigue, based on objective information.
Supports energy management	➤ By identifying targets for treatment; ➤ By supporting the application of recommendations, in particular those relating to activity management.
Allows monitoring of patient progress	➤ By documenting improvement over the course of intervention.

How to use the energy/activity diary effectively

➢ Take the time to thoroughly explain all sections of the energy/activity diary to the patient. It can be helpful to ask the patient to practice using the energy/activity diary by entering the information about his or her previous day (in session).

➢ Present the completed example and invite the patient to refer to it as needed.

➢ During each session, verify whether the patient has encountered difficulty filling out the diary and make sure the information is brief yet as specific as possible (e.g., avoiding vague notes such as "I didn't do much").

➢ Self-monitoring with an energy/activity diary is the first step to energy management, as it objectively documents the patient's energy management difficulties. By taking the time to collaboratively analyze the energy/activity diary at every session, this allows the patient to keep track of his or her progress and, as needed, to correct the tendency to see things in a negative light and to challenge the impression of powerlessness over his or her level of fatigue.

➢ For best results, the diary must be filled out every day for at least 1 or 2 weeks, and ideally throughout the intervention. Filling out the diary will require significant effort and motivation at first, but, as the program progresses, the patient will be able to better understand and appreciate its usefulness.

➢ Encourage the patient to fill out the diary at key times during the day (e.g., at meal times) to optimize adherence.

➢ If the patient prefers to use their own paper or electronic diary and this increases adherence to self-monitoring, this is acceptable provided that the patient provides energy/fatigue ratings throughout the day after key periods of activity.

➢ It is important to regularly (ideally each week) take a few minutes to analyze the diary together with the patient (see the "Energy/activity diary— Analysis" document in the Chapter 5).

➢ A printout of the fatigue barometer (Chapter 5) can be useful to help the patient rate their fatigue at different times of the day.

➢ Patients with greater cognitive impairment may struggle to fill out the diary. In this case it can be useful to simplify the information to note in the diary or to simplify the rating scale (e.g., use a three-level pictogram). Frequently follow up on self-monitoring.

An Essential Tool: The Energy/Activity Diary

Learning to monitor your energy and activities will help you manage your fatigue more effectively. You will be able to observe:

- ✓ **The links between your activities and your fatigue**
- ✓ **To gain a sense of control over your energy patterns**
- ✓ **To understand what activities and habits you can change**
- ✓ **To evaluate your progress throughout the intervention**

Use your energy/activity diary every day during the intervention. If you prefer using your own paper or electronic diary/planner, make sure that you rate your fatigue at key times during the day and that you take notes about your activities. Here is an example:

Date	Wednesday	→	Write down the day of the week.
Bedtime last night	10:30 p.m.	→	Write down the time you went to bed last night.
Rising time this morning	9:30 a.m.	→	Right down the time you got up.
Upon waking up this morning - Level of fatigue (1 to 5) - Activities/Meals/Naps/ Emotions	3 Slept poorly back pain Difficulty moving Didn't have breakfast	→	Rate your level of fatigue in the upper left-hand corner of each box using the following scale: **1** = I feel no fatigue, I feel energetic **2** = I feel slight fatigue **3** = I feel moderate fatigue **4** = I feel significant fatigue **5** = I feel exhausted, drained of energy
Morning - Level of fatigue (1 to 5) - Activities/Meals/Naps/ Emotions	4 Cleaned up kitchen Tax papers 10 a.m.–1 p.m. Pizza Headache	→	Write down your activities, regardless of whether or not they seem related to fatigue. Also write down your symptoms and your meals.
Afternoon - Level of fatigue (1 to 5) - Activities/Meals/Naps/ Emotions	5 Exhausted Slept from 1:30 to 3:40 p.m. Email	→	Write down your naps.
Suppertime - Level of fatigue (1 to 5) - Activities/Meals/Naps/ Emotions	4 Didn't go to my sister's because I was too tired Soup, cheese	→	Write down any social or leisure activities you missed or declined because of fatigue.
Evening - Level of fatigue (1 to 5) - Activities/Meals/Naps/ Emotions	3 television Disappointed because I didn't do much unable to finish filling out tax documents	→	Write down your emotions, impressions, or other relevant information.

Clinician guide
Presenting Basic Facts About Fatigue and Understanding the Vicious Circle of Fatigue and the Benefits of Better Energy Management

Rationale
- To normalize the patient's experience;
- To allow the patient to realize that fatigue has multiple causes, several of which can be curbed or eliminated;
- To make the patient aware that regardless of what led to the onset or worsening of fatigue (e.g., the TBI), several factors perpetuate fatigue over the long term and can be worked upon in order to improve energy level;
- To clearly understand the rationale behind the interventions suggested.

Implementation in brief
➤ Present basic education about frequency of fatigue following TBI, types of fatigue (mental, physical, general), and different factors contributing to fatigue.

➤ Present the vicious circle of fatigue:
  • Explain the illustration and verify the patient's understanding.
  • In case of difficulty with understanding, adapt language as needed, give concrete examples, or use metaphors.
  • Ask the patient to identify which elements listed in the illustration seem to connect with what he or she is experiencing.

➤ Present the positive cycle of energy management:
  • Explain the illustration and verify the patient's understanding.
  • In case of difficulty with understanding, adapt language as needed, give concrete examples, or use metaphors.
  • Discuss the patient's understanding of the positive cycle and ask the patient which elements appear to be most relevant, or which seem to hold a possibility for modifying his or her habits. (Sample questions: Can you relate to this? Do you think some things would be easier for you to change? If you had to choose one element you would like to change, which would it be?).

➢ Discuss potential impacts of fatigue:
  • Fatigue can limit a person's ability to use his or her full physical and mental potential.
  • Fatigue can influence mood and consequently impact people close to the patient.
  • Fatigue can cause a gradual decrease in certain activities. For example, some people might abandon leisure activities, decrease their level of physical activity, cancel social occasions, avoid certain household tasks, reduce their workload, or stop working altogether.
  • Being less active can deprive an individual of pleasant, relaxing, motivating, and satisfying activities. Enjoyment, relaxation, motivation, and satisfaction are in fact ingredients of energy. In other words, although some activities require energy and may seem tiring, they can also be sources of energy.

 Fatigue Following a TBI

➢ Most people who experience a traumatic brain injury (TBI) report subsequent fatigue or lack of energy.
➢ This fatigue is often felt on a daily basis, sometimes without any apparent cause, and it is not unusual for the fatigue to last several weeks, months, or even years.
➢ Fatigue is a subjective experience that is difficult to define and measure. You may feel different types of fatigue, for example physical or mental fatigue.

Physical fatigue
Difficulty sustaining a physical activity

Mental fatigue
Difficulty sustaining a mental activity

Fatigue is also distinct from sleepiness. Sleepiness is an involuntary physiological state between waking and sleeping and is characterized by the inability to stay awake and alert during the day. It is, therefore, possible to feel fatigued without being sleepy, in other words, without the body or brain being near a sleep state. If you are experiencing fatigue, it is important not to forget that although your brain injury may be one cause of your fatigue, other factors can also be involved, and some of these factors can be improved through changes in lifestyle, behavior, and ways of thinking.

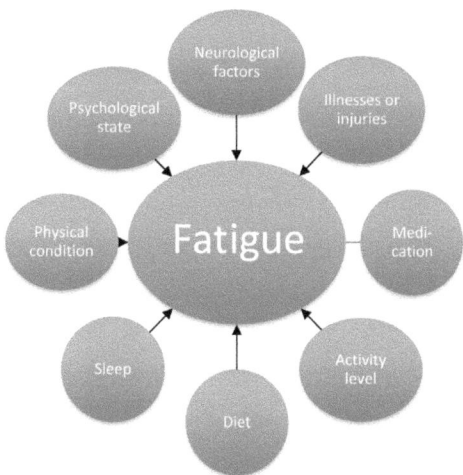

The Vicious Circle of Fatigue

When feeling tired or fatigued, it is natural to want to rest or to stop an activity for some time in order to recover strength and energy. In the short term, this strategy is appropriate. However, when fatigue is experienced over a long period of time, it can lead to an overall important decrease in certain activities: we may avoid certain situations, or even abandon certain activities altogether, therefore also losing some benefits linked to these activities, such as satisfaction, socialization, or pleasure. In the long term, not being active enough can affect our mood, our stress levels, and our sleep, because all of these aspects are linked to our activity levels. On the other hand, sometimes when we feel we have a bit of energy, we may try to get too much done and not manage our energy adequately: by overdoing, we may actually feel even more fatigued or exhausted afterward. We call this the overexertion/inactivity cycle, or the "Boom and bust" cycle. Take the time to note in which parts of this figure you recognize yourself.

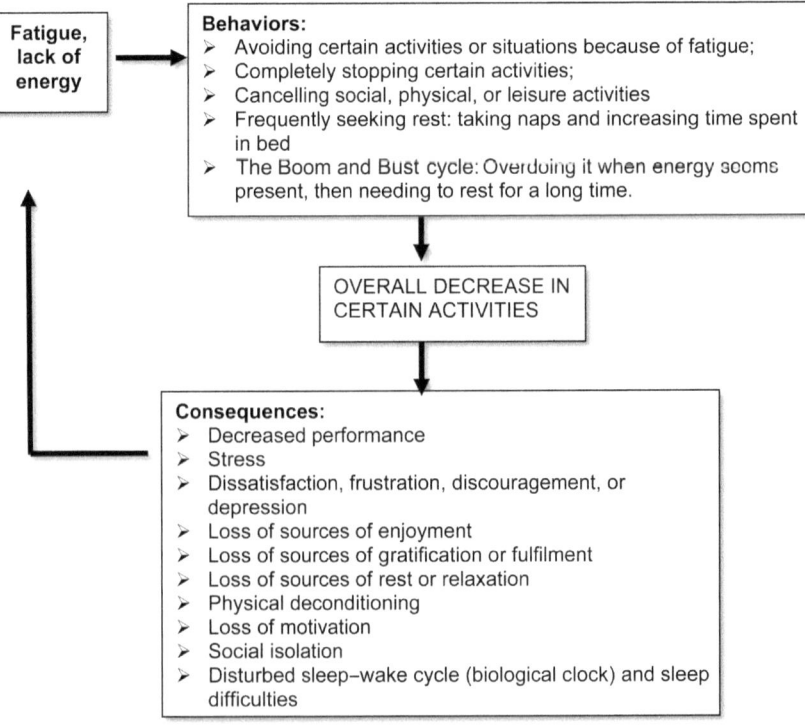

The Positive Cycle of Effective Energy Management

Effective energy management means being able to engage in various types of activities despite the presence of fatigue and while respecting your energy levels, values, and goals.

This means engaging not only a variety of activities, including your obligations, but also leisure, social, productive, or simply enjoyable things, to the level that is realistic for you at the present time. Being gradually more active will in fact renew your energy. Indeed, gradually resuming activities or trying new ones will bring you greater enjoyment, satisfaction, and self-confidence, in turn contributing to a better mood and motivation. The benefits of being more active should also extend to other areas of your life, namely, sleep, mood, physical health, and general well-being.

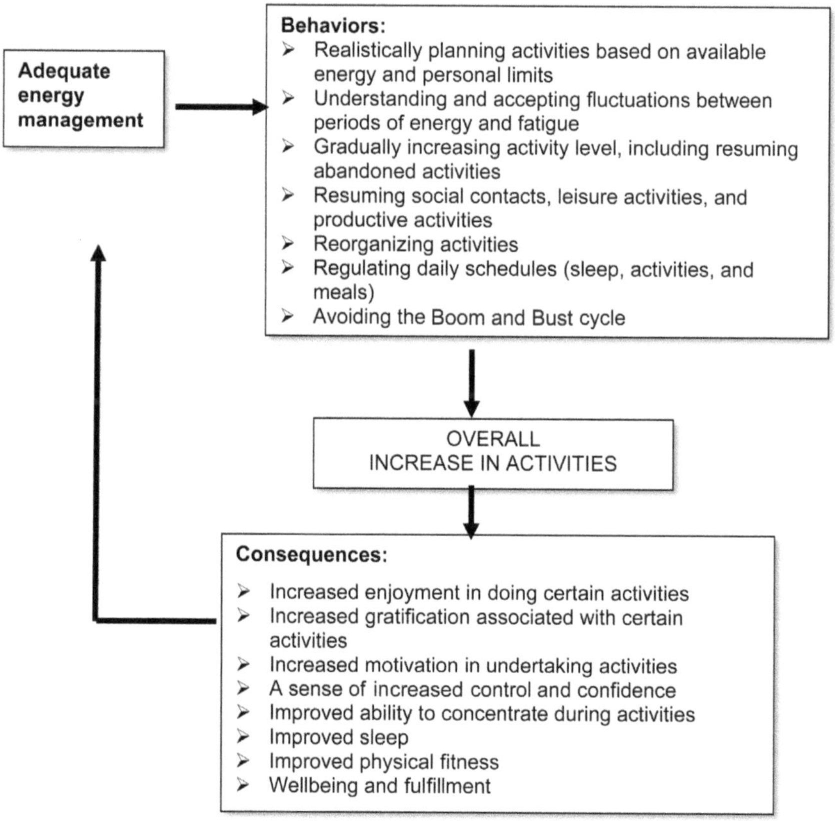

| Adequate energy management | → | **Behaviors:**
➢ Realistically planning activities based on available energy and personal limits
➢ Understanding and accepting fluctuations between periods of energy and fatigue
➢ Gradually increasing activity level, including resuming abandoned activities
➢ Resuming social contacts, leisure activities, and productive activities
➢ Reorganizing activities
➢ Regulating daily schedules (sleep, activities, and meals)
➢ Avoiding the Boom and Bust cycle |

OVERALL INCREASE IN ACTIVITIES

Consequences:

➢ Increased enjoyment in doing certain activities
➢ Increased gratification associated with certain activities
➢ Increased motivation in undertaking activities
➢ A sense of increased control and confidence
➢ Improved ability to concentrate during activities
➢ Improved sleep
➢ Improved physical fitness
➢ Wellbeing and fulfillment

Clinician guide
Understanding the Connection Between Lifestyle Habits and Fatigue

Rationale
- To inform the patient about lifestyle-related habits and environmental factors which may contribute to fatigue;
- To allow the patient to make certain changes to lifestyle habits as needed, in order to support the effectiveness of other interventions.

Implementation in brief

Review the information listed below to provide psychoeducation adapted to the patient's needs. Refer the patient to the appropriate resources if specific problems need to be dealt with (e.g., nutritionist, kinesiologist, recreational therapist, occupational therapist, or psychologist).

➤ **Hydration, diet, and substance use**

- To maintain a good energy level, it is important to ensure that the patient has a balanced diet. The energy/activity diary can provide useful information on meal numbers, times, and content. Generally poor dietary habits can influence energy level (e.g., an unbalanced or insufficiently balanced diet that is too rich in processed food, fat, sugar, salt, or starch or that is lacking in certain nutrients, such as proteins or vitamins). Direct the patient to valid information, for example, the *Canadian Food Guide* or the *Dietary Guidelines for Americans*.
- Make the patient aware of the importance of staying hydrated: inadequate hydration can significantly influence physical and cognitive abilities.
- It is important to evaluate the consumption of energy drinks or other natural products given that some of these substances contain caffeine or ingredients that have not been thoroughly tested for their side effects or can interact with other medications.

➤ **Leisure**

- Individuals with TBI often experience a decrease in leisure activities and also have less variety in their types of leisure activities, often as a result of their fatigue and other difficulties.
- Leisure activities can nevertheless bring enjoyment, satisfaction, social contacts, and physical benefits, which are all factors that contribute to optimal energy.

- It is important to invite the patient to explore leisure activities that the patient engaged in before the accident and to explore new options:
  - ○ **Reintegrating leisure activities.** Evaluate whether certain leisure activities could be adapted and thereby reintegrated into the patient's lifestyle. Together with the patient, discuss the possibility of adjusting his or her leisure-related expectations to be able to enjoy them without altogether expecting them to play out exactly as they did before the accident.
  - ○ **Exploring new leisure activities.** If physical or cognitive limitations are preventing the patient from practicing the same leisure activities as before the accident, explore his or her spheres of interest in order to find potential options to consider. Start slowly, and gradually build up while the patient progresses.

➤ **Physical activity**

- Regular physical activity is probably the intervention with most empirical support for fatigue management. Encourage exercise as much as possible and refer to the tools presented further for support.

➤ **Sleep**

- Even if the patient is not experiencing sleep problems, he or she should be reminded that good sleep habits, a regular sleep–wake schedule, and good sleep hygiene all contribute to optimizing energy level. Use the tools in the section on insomnia intervention as needed.

➤ **Posture**

- The postures adopted in various tasks or activities contribute to the amount of energy that is spent. Poor posture (e.g., a leaning or hunched-over posture) and inadequate work or personal space setup (e.g., poorly positioned keyboard, monitor, or work materials) can contribute to fatigue. Try to make the patient aware of his or her poor postures or less-than-optimal setups.
- In some cases, it can be advisable to consult an ergonomist or occupational therapist.

➤ **Stress management**

- Stress and anxiety often contribute to fatigue. Evaluate whether the patient needs support or strategies for better stress management.
- Suggest certain general strategies to help the patient manage stress, namely, physical activity, leisure, social activities, conversations with family/friends regarding his or her concerns, relaxation or breathing techniques, or psychotherapy, such as mindfulness or cognitive therapy.

 Healthy Habits to Optimize Energy

To better manage your energy, it is important to maintain healthy habits that help maintain adequate energy level.

Hydration	Drinking water regularly is important, as hydration significantly influences physical and mental capacities.
Diet	A regular and balanced diet is necessary for adequate energy. Consult the *Dietary Guidelines for Americans* or *Canada's Food Guide* as needed or make an appointment with a professional who can assist you (e.g., a nutritionist or dietician).
Leisure	Having leisure activities will increase your energy levels by providing pleasurable and satisfying moments. Try to find time for leisure activities. If you have abandoned certain leisure activities, examine how these could be adapted so as to enjoy them again, or try new ones.
Sleep and rest	Obtaining sufficient and refreshing sleep helps to ensure a good level of energy during the day. Keep to a regular sleep schedule and avoid spending too much time in bed, even if only to rest. Be sure to establish a bedtime routine, and set aside at least 1 hour before bedtime for rest and relaxation. It is also possible to rest without sleeping. You can choose activities that are less demanding physically or mentally, or that are relaxing, in order to get more energy. If you have significant sleep problems, inform your health professional.
Physical activity	Exercise is one of the best ways to renew your energy. Choose physical activities that suit you and that you enjoy, such as a sport, a workout, or simply walking. Plan regular times during the week to practice these physical activities. Choose a gradual approach to increase exercise or integrate a new physical activity.
Posture	Poor posture (e.g., leaning too much or being hunched over) can lead you to spend unnecessary energy. Be attentive to your posture and the furniture or equipment you use (e.g., chairs), especially during seated activities (e.g., working at a computer or when reading).
Stress	Stress contributes to fatigue. Keep a watchful eye on your own manifestations of stress. Eliminate stress through exercise, leisure, and social activities. Discuss your worries with the people you trust. Learn and regularly apply a breathing or relaxation technique, or listen to music to refresh your mind.

Clinician guide
Improving Self-Perception of Signs of Fatigue

Rationale
- To allow the patient to more adequately notice when fatigue is building up. After a TBI, several patients report not noticing that they are getting fatigued: they tend to continue a given activity until the symptoms become very pronounced, thus overexerting themselves. Many report that after such an episode, they "pay the price" and then feel that they need hours or days to recover. Improving patients' perception of early signs of fatigue could prevent this alternation between periods of overexertion and inactivity, also called the "Boom and Bust" cycle.
- To allow the patient to adapt his or her activities based on available energy. To do so, it can be very helpful to take some time for self-analysis.
- To be able to better identify and respect one's limitations.
- To implement energy management strategies at the appearance of the first signs of fatigue.

Implementation in brief
➤ Help the patient recognize the most common signs of fatigue, first by asking the patient about signs of his/her fatigue and allowing a free-form answer. Then use the list provided in the next tool to help structure the discussion.

➤ You might also suggest that the patient ask a family member or friend to describe his or her signs of fatigue so that the patient can compare self-perceptions with others' perceptions. However, discussing signs of fatigue with a family member or friend may cause some friction: make sure the patient is ready for this exercise, is able to adequately express his or her emotions in this context, and is receptive to hearing about how his or her fatigue is perceived by this family member or friend.

➤ You may ask the patient to be attentive to these signs the next time he or she engages in an activity that they know is demanding.

The following questions can facilitate discussion of signs of fatigue:

- What are your usual signs of fatigue?
- Are they always the same? Do they vary according to different times during the day or during different activities?
- After how much time do you begin to notice signs of fatigue when engaging in a demanding activity? Can you give an example?
- Do other people point out to you that you are starting to show fatigue? What do they notice? When they do point it out, how do you respond?
- How could you be more attentive to your signs of fatigue in order to be able to better manage your energy?

 Recognizing the Signs of Fatigue

Fatigue can manifest in different ways from one individual to another, and even at different times for the same individual. Signs of fatigue can be associated with physical functioning, behaviors and emotions, or mental functioning. It can sometimes be difficult to notice your own signs of fatigue. Using the following table, check off the signs associated with your fatigue. If you wish to do so, ask a family member or friend to help you recognize these signs.

Signs associated with physical functioning	Signs associated with emotions and behaviors	Signs associated with mental functioning
☐ Sense of heaviness ☐ Decrease in strength, endurance, or balance ☐ Pain ☐ Headaches ☐ Blank stares ☐ Less expressive facial expressions ☐ Flushed face ☐ Red, baggy eyes ☐ Change of posture ☐ Slower gestures or movements ☐ Need to move ☐ Dizziness	☐ Feeling irritable ☐ Feeling impatient ☐ Feeling more impulsive ☐ Having inappropriate reactions ☐ Feeling more aggressive ☐ Being more passive ☐ Euphoria ☐ Feeling stressed, worrying ☐ Feeling depressed or sad ☐ Feeling guilty or worthless ☐ Loss of interest or pleasure	☐ Having difficulty following a conversation ☐ Having trouble doing several things at the same time ☐ Having trouble concentrating on a task ☐ Making mistakes ☐ Forgetting things ☐ Having difficulty solving a problem ☐ Thinking more slowly ☐ Feeling in a mental fog

Other signs:_____

_____

Clinician guide
**Understanding Energy Fluctuations and the
Activity–Fatigue Connection**

Rationale
- To make the patient aware of what he or she is able to do;
- To allow the patient to be more realistic regarding fatigue and the completion of activities;
- To decrease the impression that fatigue is constantly present throughout the day;
- To develop greater awareness and objectivity about fatigue.

Implementation in brief
➤ Together with the patient, first try to draw up an inventory of typical daily activities (you may use the next tool entitled "Understanding the activity–fatigue connection"). Be sure to incorporate all of the activities noted down in the energy/activity diary. Some patients will not yet have had the opportunity to reengage in certain activities, for example, because they have not gone back to work or have not returned home. Consequently, this exercise may be repeated at different times during rehabilitation (e.g., when beginning to visit home, when returning home, and when going back to work).

➤ Use the tool entitled "Identifying sources of energy and fatigue" to invite the patient to reflect upon activities which are more or less demanding.

 Understanding the Activity–Fatigue Connection (Example)

By making an inventory of the activities you do on a regular basis, you can start to evaluate how these are related to your energy level. Here is Jean-Philippe's example:

Activity	Generally, when I do this activity:				
	1	2	3	4	5
	I don't feel tired at all	I feel slightly tired	I feel moderately tired	I feel very tired	I feel exhausted
Preparing a meal				X	
Watching a documentary on TV	X				
Having a simple conversation		X			
Filling out important forms					X
Listening to music	X				
Attending a meeting				X	
Making purchases in a store I have never been to				X	

	Generally, when I do this activity:				
	1	2	3	4	5
Activity	I don't feel tired at all	I feel slightly tired	I feel moderately tired	I feel very tired	I feel exhausted
Reading my email		X			
Writing a letter or email		X			
Mowing the lawn			X		
Following a conversation in a noisy environment				X	
Emptying the dishwasher			X		
Reading the newspaper			X		
Reading an instruction manual					X
Folding the laundry		X			
Taking a walk	X				

 Understanding the Activity–Fatigue Connection

1. Draw up an inventory of activities you typically do in a day or a week. Be sure to include activities that are recurring and/or important to you.
2. Evaluate the level of fatigue you generally feel when you engage in each of these activities.

Activity	Generally, when I do this activity:				
	1 I don't feel tired at all	**2** I feel slightly tired	**3** I feel moderately tired	**4** I feel very tired	**5** I feel exhausted

 Identifying Sources of Energy and Fatigue

The following questions are aimed at understanding the ups and downs of your energy levels. You may answer the questions at different times to see whether your answers change over time.

Identifying my sources of energy

Are there times in the day when I feel less tired?	
Which activities am I still able to do even when I feel tired?	
What are the activities that I enjoy and that do not make me feel excessively tired?	
After which activities do I generally feel relatively energetic?	
Are there activities that are restful for me?	
Are there activities that give me a sense of renewed energy?	

NOTES:

Identifying activities associated with fatigue

Are there times in the day when I feel more tired?	
Are there activities that make me feel especially tired?	
Are there activities where I tend to overdo it, for example, by doing too much or doing something for too long, and I end up extremely tired?	
What types of activities make me more fatigued? (For example, physically or mentally challenging task? Activities that require concentration or a lot of planning?)	
Do I have good and bad days (e.g., a more difficult Monday after a full weekend)?	
Are there combinations of activities that are especially tiring (e.g., demanding mental work in the morning, followed by tedious physical work in the afternoon)?	

Are there key periods when I feel especially tired (e.g., weekend home visits)?	
How could I reorganize these activities?	

Now think about what you have planned tomorrow or in a few days. Are some activities you have planned very tiring? Do you have demanding obligations coming up? Have you planned too many quite tiring activities in one day? Are they planned at a time when you will have more energy? The next exercises will help you plan these activities better.

NOTES:

Clinician guide
Countering Inactivity by Gradually Increasing Activity Level and Planning Rest Periods

Rationale
- For less active patients, to help them realize that a gradual increase in activity level may increase their energy;
- For less active patients and patients who engage in frequent overexertion—inactivity cycles, to emphasize the importance of scheduling and alternating activities and planning rest periods adequately;
- To explore alternative ways to rest rather than inactivity or sleep;
- To provide the patient with a concrete method by which to gradually increase his or her activity level.

Implementation in brief
➤ If inactivity is a major issue with the patient, start first by estimating the patient's average time spent inactive per day: inactive time includes naps, passive rest periods, passive leisure activities, such as watching television or screens.

➤ Encourage resting through relaxing activities instead of inactivity.

➤ Help patients reorganize and plan activity and rest times:
  - Work with the patient in establishing a set schedule of rest and activities. To do so, use the energy/activity diary (see "Recommendations" on the reverse) or draw up a list of potential activities and rest periods.
  - It is ideal to maintain a set rising time to foster activeness during the day. If the patient needs to get up earlier or decrease sleep time in the morning, a slight increase in fatigue may be felt in the first few days or weeks.
  - Help the patient to increase activity time for certain activities he or she is already doing successfully and help the patient plan activities that the patient will be able to reintegrate into his or her routine. Guide the patient in setting realistic short-term goals.
  - Encourage the patient to plan rest periods, to follow basic recommendations pertaining to naps, and to diversify his or her restful activities.

➤ Adjust activity time based on progress:
- Work with the patient in achieving a **very gradual** increase in time spent being active.
- During each appointment, ask the patient to evaluate the percentage of his or her success in increasing activity level using a scale from 0% to 100% (simplify this as needed according the patient's ability to evaluate his success, e.g., using a three-level scale of achievement: no success, partly successful, success).
- Encourage the patient to respect planned activity and rest periods, as well as the nature of planned activities (e.g., 15 minutes of walking, 15 minutes of household tasks, 30 minutes of reading).
- Take into account elements, such as specific illnesses or stressful events, that can explain difficulties following the established goals or schedule.

 Different Ways to Rest

Try to think of what you presently do when you feel you need a rest. You can include things, such as sleeping or lying down without doing anything.

What do I usually do when I need to rest or take a break?

- What works best and why? (circle these)
- What does not always work and why?

Now try to think of alternative ways to rest that you may want to try.
Here are some ideas:

- Getting fresh air outside after 15 minutes of a tedious task
- Going for short walk
- Sitting down (e.g., during an activity that requires standing up for long periods)
- Getting up to stretch your legs (e.g., during an activity that requires sitting for long periods)
- Having a healthy snack (e.g., fruit or warm beverage)
- Lying down on a couch without sleeping (reading, relaxing)
- Stretching or engaging in a few yoga poses
- Taking a few minutes to complete a breathing exercise or meditate
- Engaging in a relaxing activity (e.g., taking a bath, reading a good book or magazine, watching television, or listening to music)
- Engaging in a pleasant activity (e.g., calling or spending time with friends or family, chatting with a neighbor or coworker, taking a walk in an area you enjoy, or going to a cafe, restaurant, or movie theater)

Alternative ways to rest or take a break

Recommendations Concerning Naps and Rest Periods

- There is nothing inherently harmful about taking naps: a short nap can be refreshing and improve attention and alertness.
- However, some people might feel groggy for some time after a nap.
- Naps can also sometimes affect the quality of the next night of sleep: a nap that is too long or taken too late in the day (e.g., late in the afternoon or during the evening) can delay your normal sleep onset (not feeling sleepy at the usual time) or can affect the quality of your sleep (having a lighter sleep).
- To diminish the negative impact of naps on sleep, it is generally recommended to limit naps or even avoid them altogether if possible.
- If taking a nap is essential to your daily functioning or physical comfort, you do not have to give it up. However, to limit the negative effects of naps on your sleep at night, be mindful of the following recommendations.

Nap time	The best time to take a nap varies from one person to another, but the early afternoon is usually conducive to falling asleep quickly. Naps after 3 p.m. should be avoided, since they can affect sleep the following night.
Nap duration	Brief naps (15–30 minutes long) are more effective than longer naps. After a brief nap, your level of wakefulness and capacities for attention quickly come back to normal. When a nap is longer than an hour, it will likely be more difficult to wake up and it will take longer to regain alertness to be able to function. If you are unable to fall asleep in 15–20 minutes when attempting to take a nap, it is best to get up and resume your activities.
Nap location	Naps should be taken in the same environment as sleep at night, i.e., in your bed.
Substitutes for napping	Long periods of inactivity should be avoided. It is preferable to alternate between periods of activity and rest, which can be planned ahead of time or can be adjusted depending on the level of fatigue and sleepiness experienced during the day. Try to find alternative ways to deal with sleepiness or fatigue during the day, e.g., listen to music, exercise, walk outside, or engage in pleasant or social activities.

Clinician guide
**Strategies to Adapt Activities in Order to Manage Energy
Levels Effectively**

Rationale
- To teach the patient strategies that will enable him or her to better
  manage energy: simplify activities, break down activities into steps,
  planning breaks, and alternating between different types of activities;
- To help patients avoid cycles of overexertion (overly vigorous or
  prolonged activities) followed by periods of inactivity (overly passive
  or prolonged rest periods).

Implementation in brief
➤ Collaboratively with the patient examine the energy/activity diary
  and identify meaningful activities that are important for the patient
  but that he or she is not able to complete satisfactorily without
  feeling a high level of fatigue (during or after the activity).

➤ Take the time to present the different strategies in the tool entitled
  "Adapting activities to minimize fatigue."

➤ Use the energy/activity to identify activities which could be
  planned differently using the different strategies.

➤ In a new energy/activity diary, ask the patient to better plan his or
  her activities by incorporating the strategies discussed (see the
  energy/activity diary example); the patient can plan more important
  or demanding tasks during periods of the day where energy is
  generally better (often in the mornings).

➤ Ask the patient to experiment with these strategies and then review
  how things went, addressing the results and the patient's
  impressions regarding the application of strategies. It may be
  preferable to test out one strategy at a time.

➤ Suggest behavioral experiments where trial and error are allowed.

➤ Focus on building the patient's self-efficacy.

Energy management strategies	
Simplifying the activity	If the patient has been unsuccessful in completing an activity that is important, explore if planning a simpler version of the task or a simpler alternative could be envisaged. Encourage a behavioral experiment with this alternative option. The goal is for the patient to experience success and gradually test his or her ability to complete more complex or longer activities. Explore what the patient is willing to try first.
Breaking the activity down into steps	Try to find a meaningful activity for the patient as an example. Explore if the activity can be broken down into logical and manageable steps. Devise a behavioral experiment by planning different steps over several periods during the day or over several days. Assess to what extent the patient feels confident in completing the first step (if not confident enough, adjust the difficulty of the step). Assess how the patient has felt when experimenting with this strategy.
Planning breaks	Encourage the patient to plan short breaks during a demanding activity. Using the patient's specific activities that he or she needs or wants to do, find appropriate ways to take a break (sit down, talk to someone, drink a glass of water, or go outside for a few minutes). Refer or use the "Different ways to rest" tool to find effective ways to rest. If breaks are planned in advance, it may be easier to test their efficacy. Stress the importance of planning breaks before getting exhausted. Behavioral experiments may be planned to test out how much time is needed before a break becomes necessary. In this case the patient should be open to having a few more difficult "trials" in the beginning.
Alternating between different types of activities	If it is possible for the patient to alternate between different activities, suggest combining a demanding or fatiguing activity with a less demanding or more enjoyable activity, or any other activity that varies the pace. Alternating between physical and cognitive tasks may be an interesting option.

 Adapting Activities to Minimize Fatigue

Simplifying activities
- Instead of planning an overly long or demanding task (e.g., preparing a multiple-course meal), plan a simpler task that is feasible depending on your available time and energy (e.g., preparing a one-course meal).

Breaking an activity into steps
- A good strategy for better managing energy during a more tiring task is to break it down into steps.
- Make sure each individual step is not exhausting in itself. You may need to experiment with activities a few times to determine the level of fatigue you experience after each step so that you can find out how to break down the activity into ideal steps. It is best not to wait until you feel tired to stop or to change activities, but rather to stop before you even feel the signs of fatigue.
- Break the task down into logical steps.
- You may complete only one or two steps and come back to the next steps later.
- Congratulate yourself on each step achieved, no matter how small. Recognize what you have accomplished, not only what you have not.
- Put yourself in a position to ensure you will be successful: Plan longer or more complex steps for when you have adequate energy or help available. If this step is not achievable, divide it again into steps.

Example:

Dividing a task into logical steps
Task: *cooking a meal*
1. Get out required materials (5 min)
2. Rinse and prepare vegetables (10 min)
3. Cook vegetables and set them aside for later (10 min)
4. Prepare meat and cook meat (15 min)

Breaking activities down into steps

Think of two demanding activities or tasks that you either have to do or want to do in the next few days. Try to think how to break these activity or tasks down into logical steps.

Activity or task	
Step 1	
Step 2	
Step 3	
Step 4	

Activity or task	
Step 1	
Step 2	
Step 3	
Step 4	

You are now ready to plan these different steps into you energy/activity diary or weekly planner using these tips:

> ➤ **Plan breaks between steps as needed or plan less demanding or enjoyable activities after each step.** Write down your breaks and what you can do to rest!
> ➤ **Learn to accept** that an activity or task may be completed over several days for now. You will gradually learn to manage more steps or longer periods of time.
> ➤ Instead of comparing yourself to before the accident, **congratulate yourself** when each step is completed without overexerting yourself.
> ➤ **Adapt** this tool as you need: add/remove steps as you wish. Try to make it a habit of evaluating whether an activity can be divided into steps or chunks of time.
> ➤ **Note down what works best** and what does not work well.

Breaking an activity into chunks of time and planning breaks

- When you want to spend time on a demanding task, you can break it down into more manageable chunks of times.
- Plan breaks during your activity.
- Do not wait to be exhausted before taking a break: plan pauses **before becoming exhausted**.
- Identify ways to rest using a calm and/or enjoyable activity: listening to music, meditating or concentrating on your breathing, closing your eyes for a moment while remaining seated, taking a short walk, talking to someone, etc.

Tom has to prepare for an important exam:

Planning breaks
Task: *Preparing for an exam*

Study for 10 minutes
   5-minute break: listen to music
Study 15 minutes
   5-minute break: short walk
Study 15 minutes
   5-minute break: chat with a friend
Study 10 minutes

Tom congratulates himself, he has studied for 50 minutes.

Think of an activity you want to do this week that you could divide into chunks of time. Go directly into you energy/activity diary or weekly planner to plan your activity periods and your breaks.

- Be realistic in your planning: prioritize quality over quantity, and avoid overexhausting yourself.
- Pay attention to how you speak to yourself: it is far more encouraging to feel you have mastered or completed part of a task than to criticize yourself for not completing an unrealistic task.
- Plan starting important or demanding tasks at a period when you generally have more energy (e.g., around 9:00 AM if you feel more energetic in the morning).

Alternating between activities

If you have to complete a mentally or physically demanding activity, avoid spending too much time consecutively on this task. Instead, alternate between the demanding activity and an activity that is less demanding, more pleasant, differently paced, or mentally or physically less demanding. Plan manageable chunks of time as to avoid exhaustion. Here are two examples.

Mary needs to complete a mentally demanding activity: working on her tax papers. She alternates with physical tasks that are not too tiring for her.

Demanding activity	Less demanding/more enjoyable activity
10 minutes: work on tax papers	
	5 minutes: fold laundry
10 minutes: work on tax papers	
	5 minutes: put things away in the kitchen
10 minutes: work on tax papers	
	BREAK, 15 minutes: take a walk

Paul needs to do some cleaning in the house. He knows this will be very tiring. He decides to alternate with mental tasks that he also needs to do but are less demanding.

Demanding activity	Less demanding/more enjoyable activity
10 minutes: cleaning	
	5 minutes: read my mail
20 minutes: cleaning	
	5 minutes: read my email
BREAK, 10 minutes: listen to music	

Alternating between activities

Now create your own sequences. Use the following tables to alternate between a more mentally or physically demanding activity and an activity that is less demanding, more enjoyable, or differently paced (e.g., if you are doing a mentally demanding task, alternate with a physical task and vice versa).

Demanding activity	Less demanding/more enjoyable activity
Activity: How long:	
	Activity: How long:
Activity: How long:	
	Activity or Break: How long:
Activity or Break: How long:	

 **Identifying High-Risk Situations**

Selma wants to put up new curtains in several rooms of her apartment. To do so, she will need to purchase materials, take measurements, cut material, and organize her materials before sewing the curtains and making adjustments. She is unsure about where to start and knows that this is a big and exhausting project. She has been waiting to have the energy to do it. Today, she is feeling relatively good and wants to take advantage of her energy level. This is what she noted in her energy/activity diary. At each time of day, she rates her fatigue level on a scale from 0 (no fatigue) to 5 (exhausted).

- Can you identify certain activities or choices which may contribute to Selma's fatigue?
- How do you think Selma felt in the following days?

Date	Wednesday	Notes:
Bedtime last night	11:30 p.m.	
Rising time this morning	7 a.m.	
Upon waking up this morning - Level of fatigue (1 to 5) - Activities/Meals/Naps/Emotions	2 slept fairly well good breakfast	
Morning - Level of fatigue (1 to 5) - Activities/Meals/Naps/Emotions	4 10 a.m. start curtain project 11 a.m. mistakes, headache I want to finish the project	
Afternoon - Level of fatigue (1 to 5) - Activities/Meals/Naps/Emotions	5 didn't have lunch kept going until 2 p.m. but didn't finish (guilt) nap 2:30 to 4:30 p.m.	
Dinnertime - Level of fatigue (1 to 5) - Activities/Meals/Naps/Emotions	4 very irritable with children skipped yoga class too tired to make lunches	
Evening - Level of fatigue (1 to 5) - Activities/Meals/Naps/Emotions	3 TV Went to bed at 8 p.m. to try to recover	

Here are a few high-risk decisions that Selma made which led her to overexhaustion.

Date	Wednesday	
Bedtime last night	11:30 p.m.	
Rising time this morning	7 a.m.	
Upon waking up this morning - Level of fatigue (1 to 5) - Activities/Meals/Naps/ Emotions	2 **slept fairly well** **good breakfast**	💣 She initially feels energetic and wants to start her project. She feels the need to take advantage of her energy level to get as much done as possible. Her plan is probably not realistic.
Morning - Level of fatigue (1 to 5) - Activities/Meals/Naps/ Emotions	4 **10 a.m. start curtain project** **11 a.m. mistakes, headache** **I want to finish the project**	💣 She does not recognize her signs of fatigue. She does not take breaks. She has unrealistic expectations about her project.
Afternoon - Level of fatigue (1 to 5) - Activities/Meals/Naps/ Emotions	5 **didn't have lunch** **kept going until 2 p.m. but didn't finish (guilt)** **nap** **2:30 to 4:30 p.m.**	💣 She does not eat at regular times. She feels guilty and disappointed about not completing her project.
Dinnertime - Level of fatigue (1 to 5) - Activities/Meals/Naps/ Emotions	4 **very irritable with children** **skipped yoga class too tired to make lunches**	💣 Because of her fatigue, she cancels a potentially relaxing and enjoyable physical activity that could have replenished her energy. Her fatigue affects her interaction with her children.
Evening - Level of fatigue (1 to 5) - Activities/Meals/Naps/ Emotions	3 **TV** **Went to bed at 8 p.m. to try to recover**	💣 She goes to bed early with the hope to rest. However, as a result, she will spend too much time in bed : she feels tired but not necessarily sleepy, as a result she will not fall asleep easily, and her sleep is likely to be interrupted during the night. Her poor sleep quality will contribute to her fatigue the next day.

In the following days, after this particular day during which she tried to do too much, Selma feels tired and irritable and needs to limit her activities. Her interactions with her family are difficult and she misses out on several social or enjoyable occasions. **Now think about how she could have planned her day differently. What would you suggest?**

Here is how Selma could have planned her day differently using better energy management strategies.

Date	Wednesday	
Bedtime last night	11:30 p.m.	
Rising time this morning	7 a.m.	
Upon waking up this morning - Level of fatigue (1 to 5) - Activities/Meals/Naps/Emotions	☐2 **slept fairly well good breakfast**	✍ She initially feels energetic and wants to start her project. She evaluates that her project could be divided into 4 logical steps. In order to maintain realistic expectations, today she plans on completing only Steps 1 and 2: taking window measurements and preparing her material.
Morning - Level of fatigue (1 to 5) - Activities/Meals/Naps/Emotions	☐3 **10 a.m. start curtain measurements** **1o:15 a.m. music break** **11 a.m. reading break** **snack**	✍ Taking measurements is a quite physically and mentally demanding task: she decides to divide this task into manageable chunks of time and plans enjoyable breaks or alternates with a different type of activity.
Afternoon - Level of fatigue (1 to 5) - Activities/Meals/Naps/Emotions	☐3 **lunch with friend read mail or email** **PM folded laundry** **4:00-4:30 organized materials for tomorrow**	✍ She eats at regular times. She engages in a pleasant social activity. She completes Step 2 (preparing for the next steps of her project) and feels satisfied about having completed Step 1 and 2. She feels confident she will be successful completing the next steps of her project
Dinnertime - Level of fatigue (1 to 5) - Activities/Meals/Naps/Emotions	☐3 **simple dinner with children** **made lunches**	✍ Her level of fatigue does not overly affect her mood or patience.
Evening - Level of fatigue (1 to 5) - Activities/Meals/Naps/Emotions	☐3 **yoga class** **TV** **bedtime 10:30 p.m.**	✍ She engages in an enjoyable and relaxing physical activity that brings mental benefits. She maintains a regular sleep schedule.

Identify your high-risk situations
Using your energy/activity diary or your daily planner, look back on the past week. Are there situations where you could have planned your activities differently to avoid exhaustion?

Note these down:

You may have similar situations planned ahead (e.g., in the next few days). What strategy could you try among these: simplify the activity, ask for help, break down into steps, break down into smaller chunks of time, alternate between activities, and use breaks?

Situation	Strategy

Clinician guide
Promoting Attitudes and Expectations for Good Energy Management

Rationale

- To foster realistic expectations regarding current daily functioning as opposed to daily functioning before the TBI;
- To help the patient maintain a balance between various types of activities;
- To encourage the patient to reincorporate certain activities he or she has abandoned;
- To avoid feelings of dissatisfaction and lower self-esteem as a result of failing to complete activities and manage fatigue.

Implementation in brief

➤ Use the following tools in order to initiate discussion and help the patient consider adapting his or her expectations to current realities as well as asking others for help for certain activities if appropriate.

➤ For more down-to-earth patients, consider using concrete metaphors (e.g., "your battery is not as powerful as it used to be and tends to more rapidly," or "you need to keep your personal energy account from going into the red zone").

➤ Help the patient better define and maintain a balance between obligations, activities which are in line with his or her core values, and activities that could foster or better manage energy. Use the first page of the "Maintaining balance between different types of activities" tool and guide the patient in filling out the table on the second page.

➤ Encourage the patient to diversify his or her repertoire of activities by reintegrating activities that were abandoned since the TBI and that seem important to the person (by adapting them or gradually reintroducing them) and by identifying new activities based on the patient's values, interests, and abilities. Use the "Reintegrating avoided activities and integrating new activities" tool.

 Maintaining a Balance Between Different Types of Activities

Take a moment to summarize your priorities and obligations using the table below
- What is important to me?
- Which activities do I have to do?
- What needs am I obligated to meet?
- What are the activities that others expect me to do?
- How much energy do these activities require?
- Are some of these activities pleasurable?

Once you have a clearer picture of these activities, explore possibilities for change
- Do some activities take up too much time?
- Could I make room for other types of activities that could help me better manage my energy?
- What could I eliminate or delegate?
- How could I get help for certain activities?
- How could I make some obligations that are tiring more pleasurable or more manageable?
- Are there activities that I put energy into, but that are unnecessary, unpleasant, and unsatisfying? How could I eliminate them? What could be alternatives?
- Are there activities that are important to me, that are in line with my core values, but that I have put aside?
- Could I reintegrate certain activities that are important to me by adapting them or adjusting my expectations?

Use the following table to understand and then prioritize the activities on which you need to or would like to spend your energy. Keep in mind the importance of keeping a balance between necessary activities and social and leisure activities.

Activities I must do (obligations) that make me feel tired	Activities I must do, but that do not cause fatigue, or that I find pleasant or satisfying
Activities I like to do (for enjoyment, relaxation, or satisfaction) but that make me feel tired	**Activities I like to do (for enjoyment, relaxation, or satisfaction) that do not make me feel tired**

 **Maintaining Realistic Expectations About My Energy Levels**

After an accident, many people wish to "go back to normal" and expect to perform their activities at the same level or with the same results as before their injury. If this is your case, it may be helpful to adjust your goals and expectations, at least temporarily, in order to increase your sense of satisfaction and control in completing these activities.

Here are some examples of how one can adjust expectations
- Agreeing to receive someone's help to complete a task;
- Delegating a given task and accepting that it might not be done exactly the way you would have done it;
- Engaging in an activity less often or over a shorter duration, but taking full advantage of it;
- Being satisfied with more modest results or level of quality, for example:
  - ✓ Dealing with less issues simultaneously and being satisfied with the work you are able to accomplish;
  - ✓ Accepting that housework will be done a little less often;
  - ✓ Serving precooked meals once in a while if this allows you to do other, more pleasant activities.

Note down some strategies which might be useful to try:

I could accept help for these activities or tasks.	
I could adjust my expectations for these activities or tasks.	
I could do these activities less often or for less long but take full advantage of them.	

Go to your energy/activity or daily planner and note down for which activities you could try one of these strategies this week.

Reintegrating Avoided Activities and Integrating New Activities

- Are there activities that you presently avoid because they seem too tiring but that could (or used to) give you enjoyment, satisfaction, relaxation, or a sense of usefulness (e.g., sports, hobbies, or volunteer work)?
- If certain activities no longer seem possible for you since the TBI, have you considered reintegrating them in a different form, by adapting or simplifying them? Could you do these activities less often or for a shorter time, yet still find some enjoyment or satisfaction?
- How could you expand your range of potential activities?
- What new activities might you integrate into your life for greater satisfaction, enjoyment, relaxation, or well-being?
- Try talking to different people (friends, family members, or health professionals) to brainstorm different ways that important activities for you could be adapted or what new activities you could try.
- Use the following table to start your reflection

Activities that I would like to reintegrate into my life	Strategies for reintegrating these activities (examples: adapt, simplify, do less often, shorten, break down into steps, alternate with another activity, ask for help)

New activities I could integrate into my life (be creative, do not decide in advance if you will or will not like them, try them before deciding).	Strategies for integrating these activities (Plan them out? When? Where? With whom? How?)

Go to your energy/activity diary or daily planner and evaluate whether you could plan one of these activities. Start with small and realistic goals and do not expect perfection from the start.

Clinician guide
Gradually Increasing Physical Exercise

Rationale
- To take advantage of the benefits of physical activity for energy management, given that the scientific data demonstrates that a higher level of physical activity effectively decreases fatigue;
- To diversify activity types for more inactive or sedentary individuals;
- To improve physical and mental health.

Implementation in brief
➢ An evaluation of the patient's physical condition is recommended.

➢ If the patient has access to physical education or kinesiology services and sports facilities, for instance in a health-care institution, a structured program involving an assessment of baseline physical fitness and a gradual increase in physical activity is recommended.

➢ If the program is supervised by a professional, it is important to make him or her aware of the context of the TBI so that the trainer can properly adapt activities to the patient's specific needs (e.g., physical or cognitive limitations).

➢ It is advisable to set realistic goals in order to maximize the patient's commitment to his or her program of physical activity.

➢ It is essential to ensure that exercise continues beyond the rehabilitation period, for example, by identifying low-cost activities that have few environmental constraints, or by enlisting the participation of other individuals in a given form of physical exercise or in supporting the patient.

➢ When constraints are too substantial (e.g., access and cost), a walking or running program can be considered.

➢ If the patient is unable to finish a physical activity as planned, this might mean that the level is too demanding and should be decreased. Ideally, the patient should be able to finish the activity even on a "bad" day. An overly demanding is much less likely to be successful. It is essential to begin with small-scale activities and only very gradually increase their level while respecting the patient's limitations.

➢ It is important to clearly explain to the patient that practicing a regular physical activity well adapted to his or her capacities will increase energy level in the long term.

➢ A comprehensive program for gradually increasing activity level (graded exercise therapy) can be found at the following address: www.pacetrial.org/docs/get-participant-manual.pdf.

➢ Tools for applying the Canadian Physical Activity and Sedentary Behavior Guidelines can be found at the following address: www. scpe.ca/English/view.asp?x = 804.

 Increasing Physical Activity to Fight Fatigue

➤ Research shows that exercise can reduce fatigue.
➤ Even if a physical activity can seem tiring, it is important to understand that practicing a regular physical activity adapted to your abilities will increase your energy in the long term.
➤ Proper supervision (e.g., by a physical trainer or kinesiologist) can help you figure out where to start and periodically adjust your goals.
➤ A program that is too demanding or moves too fast is much less likely to be successful. Any excessive activity beyond your physical capacities is not recommended. It is essential to begin with small-scale activities and only very gradually increase their level while respecting your capacities.
➤ If you are unable to finish a physical activity as planned, then the level may be too demanding and could be decreased. Ideally, you should be able to finish the activity even on a "bad day."

Set yourself a realistic goal for every day of the week, or almost every day. According to the World Health Organization, in total during the week, an adult should aim for:

- ○ at least **150 minutes of moderate-intensity** aerobic physical activity the week
- ○ at least **75 minutes of vigorous-intensity** aerobic physical activity or an equivalent **combination** of moderate- and vigorous-intensity activity

---

Note down any ideas you may have to increase your physical activity levels:

Try planning for this week with the following table. Then go directly into your weekly planner to place these activities.

Week of _____

	Planned activity, duration, details	Activity completed? Obstacles? Solutions?
MONDAY		
TUESDAY		
WEDNESDAY		
THURSDAY		
FRIDAY		
SATURDAY		
SUNDAY		

Set yourself a realistic goal for every day of the week, or almost every day.

Week of _____

	Planned activity, duration, details	Activity completed? Obstacles? Solutions?
MONDAY		
TUESDAY		
WEDNESDAY		
THURSDAY		
FRIDAY		
SATURDAY		
SUNDAY		

Week of_____

	Planned activity, duration, details	Activity completed? Obstacles? Solutions?
MONDAY		
TUESDAY		
WEDNESDAY		
THURSDAY		
FRIDAY		
SATURDAY		
SUNDAY		

According to the World Health Organization, in a given week, an adult should aim for a total of:
- ○ at least **150 minutes of moderate-intensity** aerobic physical activity the week
- ○ at least **75 minutes of vigorous-intensity** aerobic physical activity or an equivalent **combination** of moderate- and vigorous-intensity activity

8

Detailed Treatment Plan

OVERVIEW

This chapter provides a detailed treatment plan for an eight-session face-to-face individual intervention for patients presenting both post—traumatic brain injury (TBI) insomnia and fatigue. It combines intervention tools for insomnia and fatigue. This protocol has previously been used with some success in single-case methodology research (Ouellet & Morin, 2004, 2007) with patients with various profiles (mild-to-severe TBI, presence of cognitive limitations, some with orthopedic comorbidities). Of note, however, all of these patients had unimpaired language comprehension and expression, adequate self-awareness, and some motivation to get involved in therapy (volunteered to participate in the research). The goal of the present chapter is to present an example of treatment planning. For each session, we provide a detailed task checklist as well as associated materials (available in the previous chapters). Handouts are provided to support in-session presentation of the material and for use by patients at home. The duration of therapy and intensity of session content should of course be adapted to patient characteristics (e.g., administering the sessions over a 12-week period, splitting the material of one session into two sessions, repeating sessions with material that was not well integrated, procuring booster sessions over several months with key techniques). The authors wish to underline, however, that there is yet no research examining the efficacy of different combinations (or iterations) of these tools nor of different treatment modalities (e.g., group, self-help, and duration of treatment) or other adaptations.

For more information:

Ouellet, M-C., & Morin, C.M. (2007). Efficacy of cognitive-behavioral therapy for insomnia associated with traumatic brain injury: A single-case experimental design. *Archives of Physical Medicine and Rehabilitation, 88*, 1581–1592.

Ouellet, M-C., & Morin, C.M. (2004). Cognitive-behavioral therapy for the management of insomnia associated with traumatic brain injury: a case study. *Archives of Physical Medicine and Rehabilitation, 5*, 1298–1302.

Overview of Treatment Session Outlines

Session	Content
1	• Establishing alliance • Overview of the treatment • Presentation of importance of self-monitoring and support from significant other • Psychoeducation on sleep and insomnia (and impacts of TBI on sleep) • Review of sleep diary
2	• Review of sleep diary (and address any concerns regarding self-monitoring) • Introduction to stimulus control procedures • Introduction to sleep restriction procedures
3	• Review of sleep diary; adjustment of sleep window • Review of stimulus control and sleep restriction procedures • Review of problems encountered during implementation of stimulus control and sleep restriction • Presentation of sleep hygiene recommendations • Presentation of rationale and strategies for increasing physical activity
4	• Review of sleep diary; adjustment of sleep window • Continuation of stimulus control and sleep restriction procedures • Introduction to brief cognitive therapy for insomnia
5	• Review of sleep diary; adjustment of sleep window • Follow-up on behavioral strategies: stimulus control and sleep restriction procedures • Follow-up on brief cognitive therapy • Introduction to self-monitoring for fatigue (energy/activity diary) • Psychoeducation on fatigue
6	• Review of sleep diary; adjustment of sleep window • Follow-up on behavioral strategies: stimulus control and sleep restriction procedures • Presentation of sleep hygiene recommendations • Review of fatigue diary • Presentation of energy/activity management skills training
7	• Review of sleep diary; adjustment of sleep window • Follow-up on behavioral strategies: stimulus control and sleep restriction procedures • Review of energy/activity diary • Continuation of fatigue management skills training
8	• Review of sleep diary; adjustment of sleep window • Review of progress and learning • Maintenance of treatment gains and prevention of relapse

Treatment Session 1

Session tasks

- ❏ 1. Set agenda
- ❏ 2. Inquire about patient's goals and expectations (adjust any unrealistic goals/expectations) and foster collaboration
- ❏ 3. Self-management approach: collaborative relationship, effort and commitment, importance of between session works (at-home action plans), importance of getting the support from a significant throughout the treatment period
- ❏ 4. Treatment overview
- ❏   4.1. Structure: number and duration of sessions, establish housekeeping rules
- ❏   4.2. Behavioral components: focus on habits and schedules
- ❏   4.3. Cognitive components: focus on attitudes and beliefs
- ❏   4.4. Educational components: information on sleep, insomnia, energy, fatigue, and healthy lifestyle
- ❏ 5. Presenting the importance of self-monitoring with the sleep diary
- ❏   5.1. Review sleep diary (address compliance, clarify unclear information)
- ❏   5.2. Explain the rationale and benefits of using the sleep diary
- ❏ 6. Psychoeducation: basic information on insomnia
- ❏   6.1. Information on sleep following traumatic brain injury
- ❏   6.2. Information on the definition, prevalence, impact, and risk factors of insomnia
- ❏   6.3. Information on the development of insomnia
- ❏   6.3.1. Presentation of the three types of contributing factors (predisposing, precipitating, and perpetuating factors)
- ❏   6.3.2. Focus on perpetuating factors
- ❏   6.3.3. Adaptation of the model to the patient's sleep problem
- ❏ 7. Psychoeducation: basic information on sleep
- ❏   7.1. Information on the main mechanisms involved in the sleep–wake cycle (sleep drive and biological clock)
- ❏   7.2. Information on sleep stages and cycles
- ❏ 8. Summary and at-home action plan
- ❏   8.1. Self-monitoring with the sleep diary
- ❏   8.2. Read handouts and note any questions for next session

Materials for Session 1

Assessment Tools	• Sleep diary (full or short version) • Sleep diary—Example and instructions • Sleep diary—Analysis • Sleep diary—How to compute sleep efficiency?
Clinician Guides	• Establishing effective self-monitoring with the sleep diary • Presenting basic information on insomnia • Presenting basic information on sleep
Patient Handouts	• Self-management of insomnia • An essential tool: the sleep diary • Sleep following a traumatic brain injury • What is chronic insomnia and how common is it? • What causes insomnia? • Factors which perpetuate insomnia • How sleep is produced • Stages of sleep and sleep cycles • Helping a family member or friend manage insomnia (for significant others)

Note: Introducing the self-management approach, presenting self-monitoring, and securing support from a significant other are the three essential goals of the first treatment session. It is necessary to ensure that the participant understands and adheres to these elements. As the time taken to cover this content may different across individuals, basic information on insomnia and sleep may need to be postponed and could then be covered in later sessions (e.g., during Sessions 2 and 3). Sleep diaries can be printed out for the entire duration of the intervention or sent to patients by email.

Treatment Session 2

Session tasks

- ❑   1. Set agenda
- ❑   2. Review of sleep diary; address any concerns regarding self-monitoring
- ❑   3. Introduction of restriction of time in bed: limiting the time spent in bed to actual sleeping time
- ❑   3.1. Present rationale and explain how the sleep window will be set and adjusted
- ❑   3.2. Review sleep diary and set initial sleep window
- ❑   3.3. Plan for initial setbacks
- ❑   4. Present rationale of each stimulus control recommendation and insist on application of all recommendations
- ❑   4.1. Set aside at least one hour before bedtime for rest and relaxation
- ❑   4.2. Go to bed only when sleepy
- ❑   4.3. Get out of bed when unable to sleep within 15–20 min
- ❑   4.4. Get out of bed at the same time every morning
- ❑   4.5. Reserve the bed and bedroom for sleep
- ❑   4.6. Limit naps during the day
- ❑   4.7. Plan for setbacks and inform significant others
- ❑   5. Summary and at-home action plan
- ❑   5.1. Self-monitoring with the sleep diary (identify any difficulty)
- ❑   5.2. Apply restriction of time in bed daily (sleep window)
- ❑   5.3. Apply all stimulus control procedures
- ❑   5.4. Discuss behavioral strategies for insomnia with significant other to get support (provide handout)
- ❑   5.5. Read handouts and note any questions for next session

Materials for Session 2

Clinician Guides	• Restriction of time in bed: limiting the time spent in bed to actual sleeping time • Stimulus control: recreating a time and place for sleep • Motivational strategies when encountering resistance • Clinical challenges and solutions to adapt CBT to the context of TBI
Patient Handouts	• Limiting the time spent in bed to actual sleeping time • Recreating a time and place for sleep • Helping a family member or friend manage insomnia (for significant others)

Treatment Session 3

Session tasks

❑   1. Set agenda
❑   2. Review of sleep diary
❑   3. Review of restriction of time in bed
❑   3.1. Evaluate compliance with initial recommended sleep window
❑   3.2. Identify methods to enhance compliance
❑   3.2.1. Find activities to stay awake until prescribed bedtime
❑   3.2.2. Find activities to increase motivation to get out of bed in the morning
❑   3.2.3. Use alarm clock to maintain regular rising time
❑   3.3. Review rationale using behavioral model
❑   3.4. Set new sleep window based on sleep diary
❑   4. Review of stimulus control
❑   4.1. Review rationale using behavioral model
❑   4.2. Review all procedures
❑   4.3. Identify methods to enhance compliance
❑   4.3.1. Find activities to engage in when getting out of bed in the middle of the night
❑   4.3.2. Identify behavioral cues of sleepiness
❑   4.3.3. Find activities to fight sleepiness at inappropriate times
❑   4.3.4. Secure support from spouse/significant others
❑   4.3.5. Use alarm clock to maintain regular rising time
❑   5. Presentation of sleep hygiene recommendations
❑   6. Summary and at-home action plan
❑   6.1. Apply restriction of time in bed and stimulus control procedures
❑   6.2. Self-monitoring with the sleep diary (identify any difficulty)

Materials for Session 3

Clinician Guides	• Restriction of time in bed: limiting the time spent in bed to actual sleeping time • Stimulus control: recreating a time and place for sleep • Presenting basic information on sleep hygiene • Gradually increasing physical activity to better manage fatigue • Motivational strategies when encountering resistance • Clinical challenges and solutions to adapt CBT to the context of TBI
Patient Handouts	• Limiting the time spent in bed to actual sleeping time • Recreating a time and place for sleep • Sleep hygiene: maintaining lifestyle habits that promote good sleep • Increasing physical activity to fight fatigue

Treatment Session 4

Session tasks

- ❏   1. Set agenda
- ❏   2. Review of sleep diary
- ❏   3. Review of restriction of time in bed (set sleep window) and stimulus control
- ❏   4. Introduction to brief cognitive therapy for insomnia
- ❏   4.1. Administer the Dysfunctional Beliefs and Attitudes about Sleep Scale (or use scale previously completed during Assessment)
- ❏   4.2. Identify and discuss beliefs and attitudes that perpetuate insomnia, and alternatives that promote sleep
- ❏   4.2.1. Maintain realistic expectations toward sleep
- ❏   4.2.2. Do not try to force sleep
- ❏   4.2.3. Review the causes of insomnia
- ❏   4.2.4. Avoid giving sleep too much importance
- ❏   4.2.5. Avoid blowing the consequences of sleep difficulties out of proportion
- ❏   4.2.6. Develop a tolerance for variations in sleep
- ❏   4.2.7. Avoid comparing your sleep to what it was before the injury
- ❏   4.3. Present strategies for better management of worries during the evening and at night
- ❏   5. Summary and at-home action plan
- ❏   5.1. Experiment with strategies to manage worries
- ❏   5.2. Focus on beliefs and attitudes promoting good sleep
- ❏   5.3. Read handouts and note any questions for next session
- ❏   5.4. Apply restriction of time in bed and stimulus control procedures

Materials for Session 4

Assessment tools	• Dysfunctional Beliefs and Attitudes about Sleep Scale
Clinician Guides	• Brief cognitive therapy: promoting beliefs and attitudes that are conducive to sleep and helping to manage worries
Patient Handouts	• Beliefs and attitudes that promote good sleep • Strategies for better management of worries when going to bed or during nighttime awakenings

Treatment Session 5

Session tasks

❑ 1. Set agenda
❑ 2. Review of sleep diary
❑ 3. Review of restriction of time in bed (set sleep window) and stimulus control
❑ 4. Review of cognitive strategies for insomnia
❑   4.1. Beliefs and attitudes promoting good sleep
❑   4.2. Strategies to manage worries at night
❑ 5. Psychoeducation on fatigue—Part 1
❑   5.1. Provide information on fatigue following traumatic brain injury
❑   5.2. Present of the vicious circle of fatigue and the benefits of the positive cycle of energy management
❑ 6. Introduction to self-monitoring for fatigue with the daytime energy diary
❑   6.1. Review energy/activity diary (encourage compliance, clarify unclear data)
❑   6.2. Explain the rationale and benefits of using the energy diary
❑ 7. Summary and at-home action plan
❑   7.1. Focus on self-monitoring of energy level and activities
❑   7.2. Read handouts and note any questions for next session
❑   7.3. Discuss behavioral strategies for fatigue with significant other to get support (provide handout)
❑   7.4. Apply restriction of time in bed, stimulus control procedures, beliefs and attitudes that promote good sleep, and strategies to manage worries

Materials for Session 5

Assessment Tools	<ul><li>Energy/Activity Diary</li><li>Energy/Activity Diary—Example and instructions</li><li>Energy/Activity Diary—Analysis</li></ul>
Clinician Guides	<ul><li>Establishing effective self-monitoring with the energy/activity diary</li><li>Motivational strategies when encountering resistance</li><li>Clinical challenges and solutions to adapt CBT to the context of TBI</li></ul>
Patient Handouts	<ul><li>Self-management of energy and fatigue</li><li>An essential tool: the energy/activity diary</li><li>Fatigue following a traumatic brain injury</li><li>The vicious circle of fatigue</li><li>The positive cycle of effective energy management</li></ul>

Treatment Session 6

Session tasks

❑   1. Set agenda
❑   2. Review of sleep diary and energy diary; address any issues with completion and compliance
❑   3. Review of restriction of time in bed (set sleep window) and stimulus control
❑   4. Review of cognitive strategies for insomnia
❑   5. Presentation of sleep hygiene recommendations
❑   6. Psychoeducation on fatigue—Part 2
❑   6.1. Understanding the links between lifestyle habits and fatigue
❑   6.2. Improving self-perception of signs of fatigue
❑   6.3. Understanding energy level fluctuations and the activity—fatigue connection
❑   7. Summary and at-home action plan
❑   7.1. Focus on identifying the signs of fatigue
❑   7.2. Identification of sources of energy and sources of fatigue
❑   7.3. Read handouts and note any questions for next session
❑   7.4. Apply restriction of time in bed, stimulus control procedures, beliefs and attitudes that promote good sleep, strategies to manage worries, and sleep hygiene recommendations

Materials for Session 6

Clinician Guides	• Presenting basic facts about fatigue and understanding the vicious circle of fatigue and the benefits of better energy management • Understanding the connection between lifestyle habits and fatigue • Improving self-perception of signs of fatigue • Understanding energy level fluctuations and the activity–fatigue connection
Patient Handouts	• Healthy habits to optimize energy • Recognizing the signs of fatigue • Understanding the activity–fatigue connection (example) • Identifying sources of energy and fatigue

Treatment Session 7

Session tasks

- ❏ 1. Set agenda
- ❏ 2. Review of sleep diary and energy diary
- ❏ 3. Review of restriction of time in bed (set sleep window) and stimulus control
- ❏ 4. Review of cognitive strategies for insomnia
- ❏ 5. Review of sleep hygiene recommendations
- ❏ 6. Present fatigue/energy management strategies
- ❏   6.1. Gradually increasing activity level, physical activity
- ❏   6.2. Planning rest periods
- ❏   6.3. Adapting activities to minimize fatigue
- ❏   6.4. Promoting attitudes and expectations for good energy management
- ❏ 7. Summary and at-home action plan
- ❏   7.1. Focus on increasing activity level (including physical activity)
- ❏   7.2. Identify targets to maintain a balance between types of activities
- ❏   7.3. Identify activities to adapt, reintegrate, or integrate
- ❏   7.4. Read handouts and note any questions for next session
- ❏   7.5. Apply restriction of time in bed, stimulus control procedures, beliefs and attitudes that promote good sleep, strategies to manage worries, and sleep hygiene recommendations

Materials for Session 7

Clinician Guides	• Counteracting inactivity by gradually increasing activity level and planning rest periods • Strategies to adapt activities in order to manage energy levels effectively • Promoting attitudes and expectations for good energy management • Motivational strategies when encountering resistance • Clinical challenges and solutions to adapt CBT to the context of TBI
Patient Handouts	• Different ways to rest • Recommendations concerning naps and rest periods • Adapting activities to minimize fatigue • Identifying high-risk situations • Maintaining a balance between different types of activities • Reintegrating avoided activities and integrating new activities • Maintaining realistic expectations about my energy levels • Helping a family member or friend manage fatigue (for significant others)

Treatment Session 8

Session tasks

- ❏ 1. Set agenda
- ❏ 2. Review of sleep diary and energy diary
- ❏ 3. Review of restriction of time in bed (set sleep window) and stimulus control
- ❏ 4. Review of cognitive strategies for insomnia
- ❏ 5. Review of sleep hygiene recommendations
- ❏ 6. Review of fatigue management skills training
- ❏ 7. Evaluate treatment progress and goal attainment
- ❏   7.1. Review progress with charts
- ❏   7.2. Compare goal attainment to initial expectations
- ❏   7.3. Provide feedback regarding progress and compliance with behavioral procedures
- ❏   7.4. Emphasize specific problem areas needing more attention
- ❏ 8. Relapse prevention
- ❏   8.1. Make distinction between lapse and relapse
- ❏   8.2. Discuss the inevitability of occasional poor nights or periods of fatigue
- ❏   8.3. Identify high-risk situations and potential strategies
- ❏   8.4. Give tips for coping with future setbacks
- ❏ 9. Summary and closure
- ❏ 10. Consider and plan booster sessions as needed

Index

Note: Page numbers followed by "*f*" and "*t*" refer to figures and tables, respectively.

A

Abdominal breathing, 206
Actigraphs, 72
Actigraphy, 72
Activity, 235–237
  activity–fatigue connection, 234–237
  management for fatigue, 92–93
Acupuncture, 28
Adherence, issues with, 101–102
Alcohol, 64, 180*t*
Anosognosia, 7
Anxiety, 228–230
  disorders, 10, 65
  symptoms of, 101
APOE e4 genotype, 30–31
Assessment of insomnia and fatigue, 61–72
  clinical interviews, 66–67
  diaries, 67–70
  habitual sleep–wake schedule, 63–64
  history, nature, and manifestations, 62
  lifestyle and environmental factors, 64
  medications and treatments, 64
  objective measures, 71–72
  patients' readiness for intervention,
    72–74
  questionnaires, 70–71
  screening for psychopathology, 65
  screening for sleep disorders, 65
  symptoms on evolution of brain injury
    condition/adaptation, 63
  tools, 74
Assessment tools for post–TBI insomnia,
  107
  case conceptualization summary,
    135–136
  clinical interview on insomnia following
    TBI, 109–119
  DBAS, 129–134
  DSM-5 diagnostic criteria for insomnia
    disorder, 108

ISI, 126–127
  scoring and interpretation, 128
  sleep diary, 120–122
    analysis, 123
  sleep efficiency, 124–125
Attitudes, 94–95, 200–203
Average sleep time, 195

B

Barrow Neurological Institute Fatigue
  Scale, 70–71
Bedtime restriction, 24, 189–193
  limiting the time spent in bed to actual
    sleeping time, 194–197
Behavioral
  particularities for TBI, 99
  and personality changes for TBI, 9
  strategies, 179
Beliefs and attitudes, in promoting good
  sleep, 200–203
Benzodiazepine receptor agonists, 22
Biological clock, 176–177
"Boom and Bust cycle", 37, 40, 91
Breathing strategies, 206

C

Caffeine, 64, 83, 180*t*
Cannabis, 64
Caregivers, 11–12
CBT. *See* Cognitive–behavioral therapy
  (CBT)
Cerebral atrophy, 4
Chronic fatigue syndrome (CFS), 38
Chronic insomnia, 171
Circadian clock, 176–177
Clinical interviews, 66–67
  on insomnia following TBI, 109–119
  post–TBI fatigue interview, 67
  post–TBI insomnia interview, 66–67

Cognitive and behavioral strategies, 39–40
Cognitive fatigability, 90–91
Cognitive impairments for TBI, 8–9, 98–99
Cognitive therapy, 198. *See also*
    Cognitive–behavioral therapy (CBT)
  beliefs and attitudes for promoting good
    sleep, 200–203
  for insomnia, 24, 87–89
  motivating activities, 199
  strategies for better management of
    worries, 204–206
Cognitive-behavioral interventions, 159,
    213–214
Cognitive–behavioral therapy (CBT),
    23–28, 77. *See also* Traumatic brain
    injury (TBI)
  components
    for post–TBI insomnia, 82–89
    specific to post–TBI fatigue, 90–95
  effective self-monitoring, 79–82
  graded physical exercise, 95–96
  self-management approach, fostering,
    77–78
  stress and worry management, 96
  treatment components, 77–82
"Constructive worry" technique, 26–27
Coping hypothesis, 31
"Coup and/or contrecoup" forces, 4
Course
  chronic, 19–20, 90–91
  fatigue, 34
Cross-lagged analysis, 33

D
Daily activities, 11
Daytime
  napping, 63–64
  polysomnography, 72
  sleepiness, 33, 162
DBAS. *See* Dysfunctional beliefs and
    attitudes about sleep (DBAS)
Deep sleep, 178
Depression symptoms, 101
Diagnostic and Statistical Manual of Mental
    Disorders (DSM)
  diagnostic criteria for insomnia disorder,
    107–108
  DSM-IV, 14
Diaries, 67–70
  energy/activity diary, 69–70, 81–82, 143,
    219–222
  sleep diary, 68–69

Diet, 228–231
Diffuse axonal injury, 4
Disability, post–TBI fatigue, 32–33
Discrete assessment, 61–62
Dysfunctional beliefs and attitudes about
    sleep (DBAS), 88–89, 107, 129–134

E
Early morning awakening (EMA), 69
ED. *See* Emergency department (ED)
Education about health-related habits and
    environment, 38
EMA. *See* Early morning awakening (EMA)
Emergency department (ED), 3
Energy
  fluctuations, 234
    identifying sources of energy and
      fatigue, 238–240
  healthy habits to optimize, 230
  levels, 260
  self-management of, 215–216
Energy management, 223–224
  positive cycle of, 227
  promoting attitudes and expectations for,
    257
    maintaining a balance between
      different types of activities, 258–259
    maintaining realistic expectations, 260
    reintegrating avoided activities and
      integrating new activities, 261–262
  strategies to adapt activities, 246–247
    adapting activities to minimize fatigue,
      248–252
    identifying high-risk situations, 253–256
Energy/activity diary, 69–70, 81–82, 143,
    219–222
  analysis, 146
  example and instructions, 145
Excessive sleepiness, 72
Exercise, post–TBI fatigue, 38

F
Family
  caregivers, 11–12
  member involvement, 96–98
Fatigability, 29
Fatigue, 12–13, 217–218
  assessment, 61–72
  barometer, 69–70, 153
  countering inactivity by gradually
    increasing activity level, 241–242

recommendations concerning naps and rest periods, 245
different ways to rest, 243–244
diagnostic criteria for TBI-related fatigue, 138
dimensions, 70–71
energy fluctuations and activity, 234
gradually increasing physical exercise, 263–264
improving self-perception of signs of fatigue, 231–232
signs of fatigue, recognizing, 233
increasing physical activity to fight fatigue, 265–267
interaction between insomnia and, 40–41
intervention strategies for post-TBI fatigue, 213–214
lifestyle habits and, 228–229
management module, 40
numerical rating scale, 152
positive cycle of effective energy management, 227
promoting attitudes and expectations for energy management, 257
self-monitoring establishment with energy/activity diary, 219–220
versus sleepiness, 33
strategies to adapt activities, 246–247
understanding connection between lifestyle habits and, 228–229
and vicious circle of fatigue, 223–224, 226
Fatigue Impact Scale, 70–71
Fatigue severity scale (FSS), 70–71, 150
scoring and interpretation, 151

G
Gastrointestinal condition, 65
General fatigue, 70–71
Glasgow Coma Scale, 4–5
Global Fatigue Index, 70–71
Graded physical exercise, 95–96

H
Healthy habits to optimize energy, 230
Hydration, 228–231
Hypersomnia, 12
Hypnogram, 71–72
Hypnotic drugs, 22

I
Insomnia, 12, 14, 21, 162
assessment, 61–72
clinical challenges and solutions to adapt CBT for insomnia, 208–209
cognitive therapy for, 87–89
helping a family member or friend for management of, 162–163
interaction between fatigue and, 40–41
presenting basic information on, 169
causes of insomnia, 172
chronic insomnia, 171
factors perpetuating insomnia, 173–174
sleep following traumatic brain injury, 170
psychoeducation about, 82
working on unhelpful thoughts, beliefs, and attitudes about sleep, 87–89
Insomnia Severity Index (ISI), 70, 107, 126–127
scoring and interpretation, 128
Intervention strategies
for post-TBI fatigue, 213–214
helping family member or friend manage fatigue, 217–218
self-management of energy, 215–216
for post-TBI insomnia, 159
Interviews
post–TBI fatigue, 67
post–TBI insomnia, 66–67
ISI. See Insomnia Severity Index (ISI)

L
Leisure activities, 228–231
Lifestyle habits and fatigue, 228–229
healthy habits to optimize energy, 230
Light sleep, 178
Light therapy, 39

M
Maintenance of Wakefulness Test, 72
Major depression, 65
Medication for post–TBI insomnia, 16
Mental fatigue, 29, 70–71
Mentally demanding activity, 251
MFI. See Multidimensional Fatigue Inventory (MFI)
Mild traumatic brain injury (Mild TBI), 5–6, 21, 34
Mindfulness-based techniques, 24

Moderate-to-severe TBI, 7, 21
Mood, post–TBI fatigue, 32–33
Motivation(al)
  impact of fatigue on, 70–71
  interviewing techniques, 78
  issues with, 101–102
  strategies, 207
Multidimensional Fatigue Inventory (MFI), 34, 35f, 70–71, 147
  scoring and interpretation, 148–149
Multiple Sleep Latency Test, 72

N
Naps, 86
Narcolepsy, 15–16, 65
National Institute for Clinical Excellence (NICE), 39–40
Nicotine, 64, 180t
Nighttime polysomnography, 71–72
Normal sleep, psychoeducation about, 82

P
"Pacing" for fatigue, 92–93
Pain and post–TBI
  fatigue, 32–33
  insomnia, 16–17
Parasomnias, 65
Perceptions of fatigue, 94
Periodic leg movements, 65
Physical activity, 228–231
Physical exercise, gradual increase of, 263–264
Physical fatigue, 70–71
Physical impairment for TBI, 100
Pittsburgh Sleep Quality Index (PSQI), 21, 23, 70
Polypharmacy, 100
Polysomnography (PSG), 71
Post–traumatic brain injury fatigue, 12, 29–40
  case conceptualization summary for, 154–155
  clinical interview on fatigue following TBI, 139–142
  components specific to, 90–95
  energy/activity diary, 143, 145
  etiology and correlates, 30–33
    activity levels and rest, 31–32
    cooccuring issues, 32–33
    coping hypothesis, 31
    differentiating fatigue from sleepiness, 33

  pathophysiology, 30–31
  evolution and relation to TBI severity, 33–36
  fatigue barometer, 153
  fatigue numerical rating scale, 152
  FSS, 150
  interview, 67
  MFI. See Multidimensional Fatigue Inventory (MFI)
  nature, prevalence, and impacts, 29–30
  phenomenology, 36–37
  proposed diagnostic criteria for TBI-related fatigue, 138
  treatment options for, 37–40
    cognitive and behavioral strategies, 39–40
    education about health-related habits and environment, 38
    exercise, 38
    light therapy, 39
    pharmacological treatment, 37–38
Post–TBI insomnia, 14–28
  bedtime restriction, 189–193
  CBT components for, 82–89
  clinical challenges and solutions to adapt CBT, 208–209
  cognitive therapy, 198
  distribution on scores of ISI, 20f
  establishing effective self-monitoring with sleep diary, 164–166
  etiology, 15–18
    medication, 16
    pain, 16–17
    pathophysiology, 15–16
    psychopathology and stress, 17
    sleep-related habits, 17
    traumatic brain injury severity, 18
  evolution, 18–20
  helping a family member or friend for insomnia management, 162–163
  intervention strategies, 159
  interview, 66–67
  motivational strategies when encountering resistance, 207
  nature and prevalence, 14–15
  potential impacts, 20–21
  presenting basic information
    on insomnia, 169
    on sleep, 175
    on sleep hygiene, 179
  self-management of insomnia, 160–161
  sleep diary, 167

stimulus control, 183–184
treatment options for, 22–28
    CBT, 23–28
    nonpharmacological interventions, 28
    pharmacological interventions, 22–23
Posture, 228–231
Prevalence
    post–TBI fatigue, 29–30
    post–TBI insomnia, 14–15
Problem-solving, 204–205
Prospective assessment, 61–62
PSG. See Polysomnography (PSG)
PSQI. See Pittsburgh Sleep Quality Index
    (PSQI)
Psychoeducation, 24–25, 159, 213–214
    about fatigue after TBI, and health habits
        influencing energy levels, 90–91
    about normal sleep, sleep after TBI,
        insomnia, 82
Psychopathology
    and post–TBI insomnia, 17
    screening for, 65
    TBI, 10

Q

Quality of life for TBI, 11
Questionnaires, 70–71

R

Rapid eye movement sleep (REM sleep),
    16, 178
Recreational drugs, 64
Reduction of activities, impact of fatigue
    on, 70–71
Relationship strain for TBI, 10
Relaxation, 24
    strategies, 206
REM sleep. See Rapid eye movement sleep
    (REM sleep)
Rest, for post–TBI fatigue, 31–32
Restless leg syndrome, 65
Restriction of time in bed, 83–85, 189–193
    implementation, 84–85
    rationale, 83–84
Retrospective assessment, 61–62

S

SE. See Sleep efficiency (SE)
Secondary damage, 4
Self-awareness of energy levels and signs
    of fatigue, 91–92

Self-management
    in cognitive–behavioral interventions,
        77–79
    fostering commitment and effort, 78
    implementation, 78–79
    keeping realistic goals, 79
    rationale, 77–78
    adopting scientific attitude, 79
    of energy, 215–216
    of insomnia, 160–161
Self-monitoring, 61–62
    in cognitive–behavioral interventions,
        79–82
    implementation, 80–82
    rationale, 79–80
    establishment with energy/activity diary,
        219–222
    establishment with sleep diary, 164–166
Serotonin-selective reuptake inhibitors
    (SSRIs), 16
Sleep, 228–231
    disturbances, 15–19, 32–33
    following a traumatic brain injury, 170
    medication, 100
    presenting basic information on, 175
        biological clock, 176t
        sleep cycles, 178
        sleep drive, 176t
        stages of sleep and sleep cycles, 178
    psychoeducation about sleep after TBI, 82
    recreating a time and place for, 183–188
    restriction. See Bedtime restriction
    screening for sleep disorders, 65
    sleep-related habits, 17
    sleep–wake disturbances, 12–13, 13f
    sleep–wake patterns, 18–19
Sleep and Concussion Questionnaire, 70
Sleep apnea, 65
Sleep diary, 68–69, 81, 120–122, 167
    analysis, 123
    effective self-monitoring establishment
        with, 164–166
Sleep drive, 176–177
Sleep efficiency (SE), 69, 124–125, 196–197
Sleep hygiene
    education, 24, 83
    maintaining lifestyle habits, 180–182
    presenting basic information on, 179
Sleep onset latency (SOL), 69
Sleep quality (SQ), 61–62
Sleep–wake schedule, 63–64
Sleep window, 24, 86, 190–193, 195

Sleepiness, 185–188, 225
    fatigue versus, 33
Social cognition, 8–9
Social network, 10
Social participation for TBI, 11
Socratic questioning, 24–25
SOL. *See* Sleep onset latency (SOL)
SQ. *See* Sleep quality (SQ)
SSRIs. *See* Serotonin-selective reuptake
    inhibitors (SSRIs)
Stimulus control, 24, 86–87, 183–184
    recreating a time and place for sleep,
    185–188
Stress, 17
Stress management, 96, 228*t*
Subjective self-report instruments, 70–71
Substance use, 64, 228–231

T
Time restriction, in bed. *See* Bedtime
    restriction
Total sleep time (TST), 66
Total time in bed (TIB), 69
Total wake time (TWT), 69
Traumatic brain injury (TBI), 3–13, 61, 77,
    225, 269
    behavioral and personality changes, 9
    care trajectories and prognosis and after,
    5–7

clinical challenges, 98–102
    and solutions to adapt CBT for
    insomnia, 208–209
cognitive impairments, 8–9
epidemiology, 3–5
impacts
    on caregivers, 11–12
    on daily activities, quality of life, and
    social participation, 11
physical issues, 8
psychopathology, 10
sequelae, 8–13
severity, 18
social network and relationship strain, 10
Treatment plan for post–TBI insomnia and
    fatigue, 269

V
Vicious circle of fatigue, 223–224, 226

W
Wake after sleep onset (WASO), 69
Worry management, 96

Z
Z-drugs, 22